Lecture Notes in Computer Science 9601

Commenced Publication in 1973
Founding and Former Series Editors:
Gerhard Goos, Juris Hartmanis, and Jan van Leeuwen

More information about this series at http://www.springer.com/series/7412

Bjoern Menze · Georg Langs
Albert Montillo · Michael Kelm
Henning Müller · Shaoting Zhang
Weidong Cai · Dimitris Metaxas (Eds.)

Medical Computer Vision: Algorithms for Big Data

International Workshop, MCV 2015
Held in Conjunction with MICCAI 2015
Munich, Germany, October 9, 2015
Revised Selected Papers

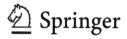 Springer

Editors

Bjoern Menze
TU München
Munich
Germany

Georg Langs
Medical University of Vienna
Wien
Austria

Albert Montillo
University of Texas Southwestern Medical
  Center
Dallas, TX
USA

Michael Kelm
Siemens AG
Erlangen
Germany

Henning Müller
University of Applied Sciences Western
  Switzerland (HES-SO)
Sierre
Switzerland

Shaoting Zhang
University of North Carolina
Charlotte
USA

Weidong Cai
University of Sydney
Sydney
Australia

Dimitris Metaxas
State University of New Jersey Rutgers
Piscataway, NJ
USA

ISSN 0302-9743   ISSN 1611-3349 (electronic)
Lecture Notes in Computer Science
ISBN 978-3-319-42015-8   ISBN 978-3-319-42016-5 (eBook)
DOI 10.1007/978-3-319-42016-5

Library of Congress Control Number: 2016946962

LNCS Sublibrary: SL6 – Image Processing, Computer Vision, Pattern Recognition, and Graphics

Printed on acid-free paper

This Springer imprint is published by Springer Nature
The registered company is Springer International Publishing AG Switzerland

Preface

This book includes articles from the 2015 MICCAI (Medical Image Computing for Computer Assisted Intervention) workshop on Medical Computer Vision (MCV) that was held on October 9, 2015, in Munich, Germany. The workshop followed up on similar events in the past years held in conjunction with MICCAI and CVPR.

The workshop obtained 22 high-quality submissions that were all reviewed by at least three external reviewers. Borderline papers were further reviewed by the organizers to obtain the most objective decisions for the final paper selection. Ten papers (45%) were accepted as oral presentations and another five as posters after the authors responded to all review comments. The review process was double-blind.

In addition to the accepted oral presentations and posters, the workshop had three invited speakers. Volker Tresp, both at Siemens and Ludwig Maximilians University of Munich, Germany, presented large-scale learning in medical applications. This covered aspects of image analysis but also the inclusion of clinical data.

Pascal Fua of EPFL, Switzerland, discussed multi-scale analysis using machine-learning techniques in the delineation of curvilinear structures. Antonio Criminisi presented a comparison of deep learning approaches with random forests and his personal experiences in working with and comparing the two approaches.

The workshop resulted in many lively discussions and showed well the current trends and tendencies in medical computer vision and how the techniques can be used in clinical work and on large data sets.

These proceedings start with a short overview of the topics that were discussed during the workshop and the discussions that took place during the sessions, followed by the one invited and 15 accepted papers of the workshop.

We would like to thank all the reviewers who helped select high-quality papers for the workshop and the authors for submitting and presenting high-quality research, all of which made MICCAI-MCV 2015 a great success. We plan to organize a similar workshop at next year's MICCAI conference in Athens.

December 2015

Bjoern Menze
Georg Langs
Henning Müller
Albert Montillo
Michael Kelm
Shaoting Zhang
Weidong Cai
Dimitris Metaxas

Organization

General Co-chairs

Bjoern Menze, Switzerland
Georg Langs, Austria
Albert Montillo, USA
Michael Kelm, Germany
Henning Müller, Switzerland
Shaoting Zhang, USA
Weidong Cai, Australia
Dimitris Metaxas, USA

Publication Chair

Henning Müller, Switzerland

International Program Committee

Allison Nobel	University of Oxford, UK
Cagatay Demiralp	Stanford University, USA
Christian Barrillot	IRISA Rennes, France
Daniel Rueckert	Imperial College London, UK
Diana Mateus	TU München, Germany
Dinggang Shen	UNC Chapel Hill, USA
Ender Konukoglu	Harvard Medical School, USA
Guorong Wu	UNC Chapel Hill, USA
Hayit Greenspan	Tel Aviv University, Israel
Hien Nguyen	Siemens, USA
Horst Bischof	TU Graz, Austria
Jan Margeta	Inria, France
Juan Iglesias	Harvard Medical School, USA
Jurgen Gall	Bonn University, Germany
Kayhan Batmanghelich	MIT, USA
Kilian Pohl	Stanford University, USA
Le Lu	NIH, USA
Lin Yang	University of Florida, USA
Luping Zhou	University of Wollongong, Australia
Marleen de Bruijne	EMC Rotterdam, The Netherlands
Matthew Blaschko	Ecole Centrale Paris, France
Matthew Toews	Harvard BWH, USA

Matthias Schneider	ETH Zurich, Switzerland
Michael Wels	Siemens Healthcare, Germany
Paul Suetens	KU Leuven, Belgium
Ron Kikinis	Harvard Medical School, USA
Ruogu Fang	Florida International University, USA
Tom Vercauteren	University College London, UK
Vasileios Zografos	TU München, Germany
Yang Song	University of Sydney, Australia
Yiqiang Zhan	Siemens, USA
Yefeng Zheng	Siemens Corporate Research, USA
Yong Xia	Northwestern Polytechnical University, China
Yong Fan	University of Pennsylvania, USA
Yue Gao	UNC Chapel Hill, USA

Sponsors

European Commission 7th Framework Programme, VISCERAL (318068).

Modeling Brain Circuitry
over a Wide Range of Scales
(Invited Paper)

Pascal Fua and Graham Knott

EPFL, 1015 Lausanne, Switzerland
Pascal.Fua@epfl.ch, Graham.Knott@epfl.ch
http://cvlab.epfl.ch/research

Abstract. We briefly review the Computer Vision techniques we have developed at EPFL to automate the analysis of Correlative Light and Electron Microscopy data. They include delineating dendritic arbors from LM imagery, segmenting organelles from EM, and combining the two into a consistent representation.

Keywords: Brain Connectivity · Microscopy · Delineation · Segmentation · Registration

Overview

If we are ever to unravel the mysteries of brain function at its most fundamental level, we will need a precise understanding of how its component neurons connect to each other. Electron Microscopes (EM) can now provide the nanometer resolution that is needed to image synapses, and therefore connections, while Light Microscopes (LM) see at the micrometer resolution required to model the 3D structure of the dendritic network. Since both the topology and the connection strength are integral parts of the brain's wiring diagram, being able to combine these two modalities is critically important.

In fact, these microscopes now routinely produce high-resolution imagery in such large quantities that the bottleneck becomes automated processing and interpretation, which is needed for such data to be exploited to its full potential.

In our work, we have therefore used correlative microscopy image stacks such as those described in Fig. 1 and we have developed approaches to automatically building the dendritic arborescence in LM stacks [5, 6], to segmenting intra-neuronal structures from EM images [1, 4], and to registering the resulting models [3]. Figure 1 depicts some of these results. In all cases, Statistical Machine Learning algorithms are key to obtaining good results. Therefore, our challenge is now to develop Domain Adaptation

---

This work was supported in part by ERC project MicroNano and in part by the Swiss National Science Foundation.

techniques that will allow us to retrain them quickly and without excessive amounts of additional annotated data when new image data is acquired [2]. For additional details on this work, we refer the interested reader to the above mentioned publications.

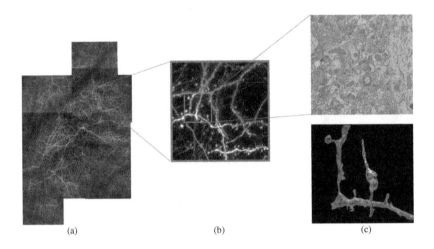

(a)   (b)   (c)

Fig. 1. Correlative Microscopy. (a) Fluorescent neurons in vivo in the adult mouse brain imaged through a cranial window. (b) Image stack at the 1 μm resolution acquired using a 2-photon microscope. (c) Image slice of a sub-volume at the 5 nm resolution above a reconstruction of a neuron, dendrite, and associated organelles.

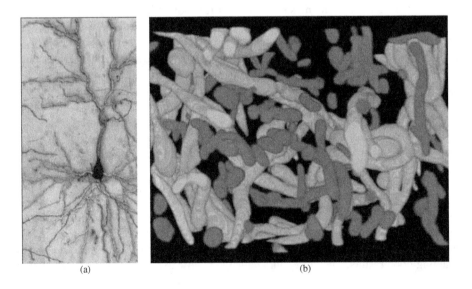

(a)   (b)

Fig. 2. Automated delineation and segmentation. (a) Dendrites from an LM Stack. (b) Mitochondria from an EM stack. The colors denote those that are either within a dendrite or an axon.

References

1. Becker, C., Ali, K., Knott, G., Fua, P.: Learning context cues for synapse segmentation. IEEE Trans. Med. Imaging (2013)
2. Becker, C., Christoudias, M., Fua, P.: Domain adaptation for microscopy imaging. IEEE Trans. Med. Imaging (2015)
3. Glowacki, P., Pinheiro, M., Turetken, E., Sznitman, R., Lebrecht, D., Holtmaat, A., Kybic, J., Fua, P.: Modeling evolving curvilinear structures in time-lapse imagery. In: Conference on Computer Vision and Pattern Recognition (2014)
4. Lucchi, A., Smith, K., Achanta, R., Knott, G., Fua, P.: Supervoxel-based segmentation of mitochondria in EM image stacks with learned shape features. IEEE Trans. Med. Imaging **31** (2), 474–486 (2012)
5. Turetken, E., Benmansour, F., Andres, B., Pfister, H., Fua, P.: Reconstructing loopy curvilinear structures using integer programming. In: Conference on Computer Vision and Pattern Recognition, June 2013
6. Turetken, E., Benmansour, F., Fua, P.: Automated reconstruction of tree structures using path classifiers and mixed integer programming. In: Conference on Computer Vision and Pattern Recognition, June 2012

Contents

Advanced Methods for Image Analysis

Poster Session

Workshop Overview

Overview of the 2015 Workshop on Medical Computer Vision — Algorithms for Big Data (MCV 2015)

Henning Müller[1,2,11](✉), Bjoern Menze[3,4], Georg Langs[5,6], Albert Montillo[7], Michael Kelm[8], Shaoting Zhang[9], Weidong Cai[10,11], and Dimitris Metaxas[12]

[1] University of Applied Sciences Western Switzerland (HES–SO), Sierre, Switzerland
henning.mueller@hevs.ch
[2] University Hospitals and University of Geneva, Geneva, Switzerland
[3] Technical University of Munich, Munich, Germany
[4] INRIA, Sophia–antipolis, France
[5] Medical University of Vienna, Vienna, Austria
[6] MIT, Cambridge, MA, USA
[7] GE Global Research, Niskayuna, USA
[8] Siemens Healthcare, Erlangen, Germany
[9] UNC Charlotte, Charlotte, USA
[10] University of Sydney, Sydney, Australia
[11] Harvard Medical School, Boston, USA
[12] Rutgers University, New Brunswick, USA

Abstract. The 2015 workshop on medical computer vision (MCV): algorithms for big data took place in Munich, Germany, in connection with MICCAI (Medical Image Computing for Computer Assisted Intervention). It is the fifth MICCAI MCV workshop after those held in 2010, 2012, 2013 and 2014 with another edition held at CVPR 2012 previously. This workshop aims at exploring the use of modern computer vision technology in tasks such as automatic segmentation and registration, localisation of anatomical features and extraction of meaningful visual features. It emphasises questions of harvesting, organising and learning from large–scale medical imaging data sets and general–purpose automatic understanding of medical images. The workshop is especially interested in modern, scalable and efficient algorithms that generalise well to previously unseen images. The strong participation in the workshop of over 80 persons shows the importance of and interest in Medical Computer Vision. This overview article describes the papers presented at the workshop as either oral presentations or posters. It also describes the three invited talks that received much attention and a very positive feedback and the general discussions that took place during workshop.

Keywords: Medical image analysis · Medical computer vision · Segmentation · Detection

© Springer International Publishing Switzerland 2016
B. Menze et al. (Eds.): MCV Workshop 2015, LNCS 9601, pp. 3–9, 2016.
DOI: 10.1007/978-3-319-42016-5_1

1   Introduction

The Medical Computer Vision workshop (MCV) took place in conjunction with MICCAI (Medical Image Computing for Computer–Assisted Interventions) on October 9, 2015 in Munich, Germany. This fifth workshop on medical computer vision was organised in connection with MICCAI after the workshops in 2010 [12], 2012 [10], 2013 [11] and 2014 [14] and an additional workshop at CVPR in 2012. The workshop received 22 submissions and ten papers were accepted as oral presentations and another 5 papers were accepted as posters. In addition to these scientific papers three invited speakers presented, linked to the main topics of the workshop, so big data and clinical data intelligence, multi–scale modelling and machine learning approaches for medical imaging with a comparison of decision forests with deep learning. All these approaches were also strongly represented at the main MICCAI conference. This article summaries the presentations and posters of the workshop and also the main discussions that took place during the sessions and the breaks. All papers are presented in the post workshop proceedings that allowed authors to include the comments that were received during the workshop into the final versions of their texts.

2   Papers Presented at the Workshop

The oral presentations were separated into four topic areas: papers on predicting disease, atlas exploitation and avoidance, machine learning–based analysis and the last session on advanced methods for image analysis.

2.1   Predicting Disease

Daianu et al. [2] identify latent factors that explain how sets of biomarkers cluster together and how the clusters significantly predict cognitive decline in Alzheimer's disease (AD). Meanwhile, to diagnose Alzheimer's with higher accuracy, Liu et al. [8] employ a multi–atlas strategy which models the relationships among the atlases and among the subjects and an ensemble AD/MCI (Mild Cognitive Impairment) classification approach.

2.2   Atlas Exploitation and Avoidance

Zografos et al. [19] present a novel atlas–free approach for simultaneous organ segmentation using a set of discriminative classifiers trained to learn the multi–scale appearance of the organs of interest. Karasawa et al. [6] in contrast present a method to segment the pancreas in contrasted abdominal CT in which only training examples with similar vascular systems to the target subject are used to build a structure–specific atlas.

2.3   Machine Learning–Based Analysis

Dvorak et al. [3] propose a convolutional neural network to form a local structure prediction approach for 3D segmentation tasks and apply it for brain tumor segmentation in MRI. Using a different machine learning strategy Wang et al. [16] develop a sequential random forest guided by voting based probability maps and apply it for the automated segmentation of cone–beam computed tomography in cases of facial deformity. Meng et al. [9] use a different random forest approach based on regression forests with added capabilities to ensure spatial smoothness and apply it to impute missing cortical thickness maps in longitudinal studies of developing infant brains.

2.4   Advanced Methods for Image Analysis

Yu et al. [17] develop an efficient image reconstruction algorithm for parallel dynamic MRI, which does not require coil sensitivity profiles and models the correlated pixel intensities across time and across coils using a joint temporal sparsity.

Krenn et al. [7] use research algorithms that were submitted in the VIS-CERAL benchmark to run them on non–annotated data sets. Label fusion of the results of challenge participants then allows to create a so–called silver corpus that has shown to be better than the best system in the competition and can be useful to train new algorithms. The approach uses relatively simple label fusion. Inoue et al. [5] use higher order graph cuts to segment the posts major muscle, a difficult structure in terms of structure contrast. The approach uses prior knowledge to estimate shapes.

2.5   Poster Session

The poster session took place during the lunch break and allowed all authors to also present their results in a poster, which is often the most adapted form to foster discussions among persons working on closely related topics.

In [1], Adeli et al. present an approach for the classification of Parkinson's disease patients using MRI data. A joint feature–sample section process is used to select the most robust subset of features leading to promising results on synthetic and real databases.

Zhang et al. [18] present an approach to multi–atlas segmentation. To solve the problem of potentially large anatomical differences between pair–wise registrations, coarse registrations are first obtained in a tree like structure to reduce the potential misalignment and improve segmentation results.

Shay et al. [15] present a new approach for the segmentation of the hippocampus in MRI infant brains. A boundary regression method is used to deal with the strong differences that infant brains have compared to adult brains.

A survey of mathematical structures for extending neurogeometry from 2D to 3D is presented in [13]. Low dose CT images are used with perfusion deconvolution.

In [4], Fang et al. present and approach to 4D hemodynamic data analysis by fusing the local anatomical structure correlation and temporal blood flow continuation. The approach limits local artefacts and leads to better results than previous approaches.

3   Invited Speakers

3.1   Volker Tresp

Volker Tresp from Siemens and LMU (Ludwig Maximilians University) Munich, Germany gave a talk about structured relational learning and the role of knowledge graphs in the capturing and representation of clinical data for large-scale learning problems. He discussed the role of tensor factorizations in the learning with graph structured data, and the possible impact on understanding, predicting, and modelling clinical events, and the large amount of linked clinical data available. The talk highlighted several aspect of big data in clinical environments and thus the topic of the workshop.

3.2   Pascal Fua

Pascal Fua of the EPFL (Ecole Polytechnique Federal de Lausanne), Switzerland presented impressive results on the use of machine learning techniques in the delineation of curvilinear structures, and reconstruction of networks such as neurons in microscopy data. Specifically he discussed approaches that overcome discontinuities and occlusions, to reconstruct a network despite imperfect data. A multi scale analysis was used.

3.3   Antonio Criminisi

The talk of Antonio Criminisi titled "Efficient Machine Learning for Medical Image Analysis" was visited by a large number of persons, as machine learning and choice of the right methods has really become a corner stone in medical imaging. Antonio is with Microsoft research in Cambridge, United Kingdom and he mentioned at the beginning of the talk that he as an expert on decision forests has taken some time to really ready into the literature on deep learning, one of the most discussed techniques in general at MICCAI 2015. He thus compared approaches of deep learning and the quite impressive performance he obtained with them but also a detailed comparison with random forests to select what technique might be best in which scenario. Random forests can in his view be reformulated as a neural network. Stability of results and also the amount of available training data were mentioned as examples to look into when choosing a technique. All applications of these techniques were on medical image analysis.

4   Discussions at the Workshop

One of the dominating topics at the conference and also at the workshop were the applied machine learning techniques and particularly the use of convolutional neural networks in various tasks of imaging such as segmentation, detection and classification. Choosing the right techniques and tools and then optimizing them is seen as a key to success.

Many people mentioned large data sets to be analysed as important for getting good results but also the challenges in getting large data sets. Multi-Centre studies and partly incomplete data sets were another topic discussed and where solutions would strongly help many of the existing techniques. Using data from several centers can create larger cohorts but standardization of imaging and meta data are challenges.

Where many data sets are now available get much annotated data with segmentations or regions of interest remains a challenge. Annotations are expensive to obtain and the tasks are often containing some subjectivity. In this context scientific challenges were highlighted as important to share data and also tools around a common objective.

5   Conclusions

Much positive feedback was given at the end of the workshop on the invited talks and the scientific presentations. The use of larger data sets and also longitudinal data were seen as important next steps. Quality ground truth and region annotations were other aspects mentioned to be important and the integration of image data with other clinical data sources to get more complete clinical analysis. Much work in medical computer vision is still required for the current challenges of quantitative medical image analysis and to bring at least a few of the tools into clinical practice in the foreseeable future.

Acknowledgments. This work was supported by the EU in the FP7 through the VISCERAL (318068) project.

References

1. Adeli-M, E., Wee, C.Y., An, L., Shi, F., Shen, D.: Joint feature-sample selection and robust classification for parkinson's disease diagnosis. In: Menze, B., Langs, G., Müller, H., Montillo, A., Kelm, M., Zhang, S., Cai, W., Metaxas, D. (eds.) MICCAI Workshop on Medical Computer Vision. LNCS, vol. 9601, pp. 127–136. Springer, Heidelberg (2015)
2. Daianu, M., Ver Steeg, G., Mezher, A., Jahanshad, N., Nir, T., Lerman, K., Prasad, G., Galstyan, A., Thompson, P.: Information-theoretic clustering of neuroimaging metrics related to cognitive decline in the elderly. In: Menze, B., Langs, G., Müller, H., Montillo, A., Kelm, M., Zhang, S., Cai, W., Metaxas, D. (eds.) MICCAI Workshop on Medical Computer Vision. LNCS, vol. 9601, pp. 13–23. Springer, Heidelberg (2015)

3. Dvorak, P., Menze, B.: Structured prediction with convolutional neural networks for multimodal brain tumor segmentation. In: Menze, B., Langs, G., Müller, H., Montillo, A., Kelm, M., Zhang, S., Cai, W., Metaxas, D. (eds.) MICCAI Workshop on Medical Computer Vision. LNCS, vol. 9601, pp. 59–71. Springer, Heidelberg (2015)

4. Fang, R., Ni, M., Huang, J., Li, Q., Li, T.: A efficient 4d non-local tensor total-variation for low-dose ct perfusion deconvolution. In: Menze, B., Langs, G., Müller, H., Montillo, A., Kelm, M., Zhang, S., Cai, W., Metaxas, D. (eds.) MICCAI Workshop on Medical Computer Vision. LNCS, vol. 9601, pp. 168–179. Springer, Heidelberg (2015)

5. Inoue, T., Kitamura, Y., Li, Y., Ito, W., Ishikawa, H.: Psoas major muscle segmentation using higher-order shape prior. In: Menze, B., Langs, G., Müller, H., Montillo, A., Kelm, M., Zhang, S., Cai, W., Metaxas, D. (eds.) MICCAI Workshop on Medical Computer Vision. LNCS, vol. 9601, pp. 116–124. Springer, Heidelberg (2015)

6. Karasawa, K., Oda, M., Mori, K., Kitasaka, T.: Structure specific atlas generation and its application to pancreas segmentation from contrasted abdominal CT volumes. In: Menze, B., Langs, G., Müller, H., Montillo, A., Kelm, M., Zhang, S., Cai, W., Metaxas, D. (eds.) MICCAI Workshop on Medical Computer Vision. LNCS, vol. 9601, pp. 47–56. Springer, Heidelberg (2015)

7. Krenn, M., Dorfer, M., Jimènez del Toro, O., Menze, B., Müller, H., Weber, M.A., Hanbury, A., Langs, G.: Creating a large-scale silver corpus from multiple algorithmic segmentations. In: Menze, B., Langs, G., Müller, H., Montillo, A., Kelm, M., Zhang, S., Cai, W., Metaxas, D. (eds.) MICCAI Workshop on Medical Computer Vision. LNCS, vol. 9601, pp. 103–115. Springer, Heidelberg (2015)

8. Liu, M., Zhang, D., Shen, D.: Relationship induced multi-atlas learning for alzheimer's disease diagnosis. In: Menze, B., Langs, G., Müller, H., Montillo, A., Kelm, M., Zhang, S., Cai, W., Metaxas, D. (eds.) MICCAI Workshop on Medical Computer Vision. LNCS, vol. 9601, pp. 24–33. Springer, Heidelberg (2015)

9. Meng, Y., Li, G., Gao, Y., Lin, W., Gilmore, J., Shen, D.: Subject-specific estimation of missing cortical thickness in dynamic developing infant brains. In: Menze, B., Langs, G., Müller, H., Montillo, A., Kelm, M., Zhang, S., Cai, W., Metaxas, D. (eds.) MICCAI Workshop on Medical Computer Vision. LNCS, vol. 9601, pp. 83–92. Springer, Heidelberg (2015)

10. Langs, G., Lu, L., Montillo, A., Tu, Z., Criminisi, A., Menze, B.H. (eds.): MCV 2012. LNCS, vol. 7766. Springer, Heidelberg (2013)

11. Menze, H.B., Langs, G., Montillo, A., Kelm, M., Müller, H., Tu, Z. (eds.): MCV 2013. LNCS, vol. 8331. Springer, Heidelberg (2014)

12. Menze, B.H., Langs, G., Tu, Z., Criminisi, A. (eds.): MICCAI-MCV 2010. LNCS, vol. 6533. Springer, Heidelberg (2010)

13. Miolane, N., Pennec, X.: A survey of mathematical structures for extending 2d neurogeometry to 3d image processing. In: Menze, B., Langs, G., Müller, H., Montillo, A., Kelm, M., Zhang, S., Cai, W., Metaxas, D. (eds.) MICCAI Workshop on Medical Computer Vision. LNCS, vol. 9601, pp. 155–167. Springer, Heidelberg (2015)

14. Müller, H., Menze, B., Langs, G., Montillo, A., Kelm, M., Zhang, S., Cai, W.T., Metaxas, D.: Overview of the 2014 workshop on medical computer vision—algorithms for big data (MCV 2014). In: Menze, B., Langs, G., Montillo, A., Kelm, M., Müller, H., Zhang, S., Cai, W.T., Metaxas, D. (eds.) MCV 2014. LNCS, vol. 8848, pp. 3–10. Springer, Heidelberg (2014)

15. Shao, Y., Gao, Y., Yang, X., Shen, D.: Hippocampus segmentation from infant brains via boundary regression. In: Menze, B., Langs, G., Müller, H., Montillo, A., Kelm, M., Zhang, S., Cai, W., Metaxas, D. (eds.) MICCAI Workshop on Medical Computer Vision. LNCS, vol. 9601, pp. 146–154. Springer, Heidelberg (2015)
16. Wang, L., Gao, Y., Shi, F., Li, G., Xia, J., Shen, D.: Automated segmentation of CBCT image with prior-guided sequential random forest. In: Menze, B., Langs, G., Müller, H., Montillo, A., Kelm, M., Zhang, S., Cai, W., Metaxas, D. (eds.) MICCAI Workshop on Medical Computer Vision. LNCS, vol. 9601, pp. 72–82. Springer, Heidelberg (2015)
17. Yu, Y., Yan, Z., Metaxas, D., Axel, L.: Calibrationless parallel dynamic mri with joint temporal sparsity. In: Menze, B., Langs, G., Müller, H., Montillo, A., Kelm, M., Zhang, S., Cai, W., Metaxas, D. (eds.) MICCAI Workshop on Medical Computer Vision. LNCS, vol. 9601, pp. 95–102. Springer, Heidelberg (2015)
18. Zhang, P., Wu, G., Gao, Y., Yap, P.T., Shen, D.: Dynamic tree-based large-deformation image registration for multi-atlas segmentation. In: Menze, B., Langs, G., Müller, H., Montillo, A., Kelm, M., Zhang, S., Cai, W., Metaxas, D. (eds.) MICCAI Workshop on Medical Computer Vision. LNCS, vol. 9601, pp. 137–145. Springer, Heidelberg (2015)
19. Zografos, V., Menze, B., Tombari, F.: Hierarchical multi-organ segmentation without registration in 3D abdominal ct images. In: Menze, B., Langs, G., Müller, H., Montillo, A., Kelm, M., Zhang, S., Cai, W., Metaxas, D. (eds.) MICCAI Workshop on Medical Computer Vision. LNCS, vol. 9601, pp. 37–46. Springer, Heidelberg (2015)

Predicting Disease

Information-Theoretic Clustering
of Neuroimaging Metrics Related to Cognitive
Decline in the Elderly

Madelaine Daianu[1,2(✉)], Greg Ver Steeg[3], Adam Mezher[1],
Neda Jahanshad[1], Talia M. Nir[1], Xiaoran Yan[2], Gautam Prasad[1],
Kristina Lerman[3], Aram Galstyan[3], and Paul M. Thompson[1,2,4]

[1] Imaging Genetics Center, Mark and Mary Stevens Institute for Neuroimaging
and Informatics, University of Southern California, Marina del Rey, CA, USA
madelaine.daianu@ini.usc.edu
[2] Department of Neurology, UCLA School of Medicine, Los Angeles, CA, USA
[3] USC Information Sciences Institute, Marina del Rey, CA, USA
[4] Departments of Neurology, Psychiatry, Radiology, Engineering, Pediatrics,
and Ophthalmology, University of Southern California, Los Angeles, CA, USA

Abstract. As Alzheimer's disease progresses, there are changes in metrics of
brain atrophy and network breakdown derived from anatomical or diffusion
MRI. Neuroimaging biomarkers of cognitive decline are crucial to identify, but
few studies have investigated how sets of biomarkers cluster in terms of the
information they provide. Here, we evaluated more than 700 frequently studied
diffusion and anatomical measures in 247 elderly participants from the
Alzheimer's Disease Neuroimaging Initiative (ADNI). We used a novel unsupervised machine learning technique - CorEx - to identify groups of measures
with high multivariate mutual information; we computed latent factors to
explain correlations among them. We visualized groups of measures discovered
by CorEx in a hierarchical structure and determined how well they predict
cognitive decline. Clusters of variables significantly predicted cognitive decline,
including measures of cortical gray matter, and correlated measures of brain
networks derived from graph theory and spectral graph theory.

Keywords: Machine learning · Diffusion weighted imaging · Brain
connectivity · Spectral graph theory · Gray matter

1 Introduction

Neuroimaging offers a broad range of predictors of cognitive decline in aging and
Alzheimer's disease, and it is vital to find out how different predictors relate to each
other, and what common and distinctive information each set of predictors provides. In
neurodegenerative conditions such as Alzheimer's disease, standard MRI techniques
can be used to detect gray and white matter loss in the brain, and fluid space expansions
that index these changes. A variant of MRI – diffusion weighted imaging (DWI) – is
increasingly used to reveal white matter microstructure abnormalities not detectable
with standard MRI. Despite the greater information available from DWI, we know far

© Springer International Publishing Switzerland 2016
B. Menze et al. (Eds.): MCV Workshop 2015, LNCS 9601, pp. 13–23, 2016.
DOI: 10.1007/978-3-319-42016-5_2

less about the microstructural changes that accompany cortical changes, and which diffusion-derived metrics change the most with disease. Recently, DWI has been added to major neuroimaging initiatives to better understand changes in white matter integrity and connectivity.

An important question in diffusion MRI is which DWI metrics best predict cognitive decline or differentiate between healthy elderly people and patients with Alzheimer's disease. It is also important to compare diffusion-derived measures to more standard anatomical measures of brain atrophy (such as gray matter volume measures); combining metrics may improve the prediction of cognitive decline. Here, we assessed a variety of DWI measures including standard ones based on the diffusion tensor – fractional anisotropy, mean, radial and axial diffusivity (FA, MD, RD and AxD). We computed these measures from 57 distinct white matter regions of interest (ROIs). We also assessed measures of brain connectivity, including network metrics (including nodal degree, efficiency, and path length, among others), and more exotic metrics from spectral graph theory – a branch of mathematics less frequently applied in the context of Alzheimer's disease [1, 2] but widely used to analyze network topology, as well as bottlenecks and information flow in graphs and networks. Brain connectivity measures describe the level of connectedness among various pairs of brain regions (such as cortical regions); these are further detailed in the *Methods* section.

We implemented a novel unsupervised *Correlation Explanation* method (called CorEx) [3–5] to construct a hierarchical network that quantitatively and visually characterizes relationships among a large set of variables. CorEx does this by learning low-dimensional representations that reflect correlations among variables. We estimated the significance of each group of DWI measures as detected by CorEx for predicting cognitive decline. To do this, we attempted to predict three widely used cognitive decline scores – (1) the Mini Mental State Examination (MMSE), (2) the Alzheimer's disease Assessment Scale-cognitive subscale (ADAS-Cog), and (3) the global Clinical Dementia Rating Sum of Boxes scores (CDR-SOB).

2   Methods

2.1   Participants and Diffusion-Weighted Brain Imaging

We analyzed diffusion-weighted images (DWI) from 247 participants scanned as part of the Alzheimer's Disease Neuroimaging Initiative (ADNI): 52 healthy controls, 29 with subjective memory complaints (SMC), 79 with early mild cognitive impairment (eMCI), 40 with late mild cognitive impairment (lMCI) and 47 with Alzheimer's disease. ADNI is a large multi-site longitudinal study to evaluate biomarkers of Alzheimer's disease at sites across North America. Table 1 shows the demographics of the participants, including age, sex, and cognitive decline scores (MMSE, ADAS-Cog, CDR-SOB) broken down by diagnosis. All participants underwent MRI scans of the brain, on 3-Tesla GE Medical Systems scanners, at 16 sites across North America. Standard anatomical T1-weighted IR-FSPGR (inverse recovery fast spoiled gradient recalled echo) sequences were collected (256×256 matrix; voxel size = $1.2 \times 1.0 \times 1.0$ mm^3; TI = 400 ms, TR = 6.984 ms; TE = 2.848 ms; flip angle = $11°$) in the same session as the

DWI (128×128 matrix; voxel size: $2.7 \times 2.7 \times 2.7$ mm^3; scan time = 9 min). 46 separate images were acquired per subject: 5 T2-weighted images with no diffusion sensitization (b_0 images) and 41 diffusion-weighted images ($b = 1000$ s/mm^2). Image preprocessing was performed as described previously in [6–8].

2.2 White Matter (WM) Tract Atlas ROI Computation

The JHU DTI atlas [9] was registered to each participant's FA map using a mutual information-based elastic registration technique [10]. Then, using nearest neighbor interpolation, we applied the deformation fields to the JHU 'Eve' WM atlas labels (http://cmrm.med.jhmi.edu/cmrm/atlas/human_data/file/AtlasExplanation2.htm) to overlay them on the individual imaging data. We calculated the average FA, MD, RD and AxD within the 52 JHU ROIs for each participant; we excluded 4 ROIs: the left and right hemisphere middle cerebellar peduncle and pontine crossing tract. These were excluded as they often fall outside of the FOV. In addition to the 52 ROIs, 5 more were computed: bilateral *genu*, body and *splenium* of the corpus callosum, the corpus callosum as a whole, and the bilateral *fornix*.

2.3 Cortical Measures

Cortical gray matter measures were extracted from the T1-weighted structural MRI scans using FreeSurfer software, version 5.3 (http://surfer.nmr.mgh.harvard.edu/) [11]. 34 cortical labels were extracted for each hemisphere from the Desikan-Killiany atlas [12]. Parcellations were reviewed for quality control and manually corrected for errors by a neuroanatomically trained image analyst. We extracted measures of gray matter volumes, surface area and thickness for each ROI.

2.4 Computing *NxN* Connectivity Matrices

To map the brain's fiber connections and create cortical connectivity networks, we combined whole-brain tractography from the DWIs with an automatically labeled set of brain regions from the high-resolution T1-weighted MRIs. To do this, we first performed tractography using Camino (http://cmic.cs.ucl.ac.uk/camino/) to recover >80,000 streamlines (below called "fibers" for simplicity) per participant, using a HARDI reconstruction scheme. During processing, we filtered out fibers less than 25 mm in length, which tend to be false positive fibers, and removed all duplicates. As described above, 68 cortical labels were automatically extracted from all aligned T1-weighted structural MRI scans using FreeSurfer, version 5.3. The resulting T1-weighted images and cortical models were linearly aligned to the space of the DWIs. The DWIs (and fiber tracts) were further elastically registered to the T1-weighted image to account for susceptibility artifacts.

For each participant, we detected the fibers connecting each pair of ROIs by considering the white matter tractography and the cortical parcellations. These were enumerated in a 68×68 connectivity matrix based on the 34 ROIs in each hemisphere;

Table 1. Demographic information from ADNI including age, cognitive decline scores (MMSE, ADAS-Cog, CDR-SOB) and sex. Here, AD stands for Alzheimer's disease.

	Controls	SMC	eMCI	lMCI	AD	Total
N	52	29	79	40	47	247
Age (mean ± SD in years)	72.4 ± 6.0	72.5 ± 4.6	71.8 ± 7.8	71.7 ± 6.8	74.6 ± 8.5	72.5 ± 7.2
MMSE (mean ± SD)	28.9 ± 1.4	28.9 ± 1.5	28.1 ± 1.5	26.9 ± 2.1	23.3 ± 1.9	27.3 ± 2.6
ADAS-Cog (mean ± SD)	5.4 ± 2.6	5.13 ± 3.1	8.0 ± 3.4	13.2 ± 4.9	20.2 ± 7.2	10.3 ± 7.1
CDR-SOB (mean ± SD)	0.0 ± 0	0.0 ± 0	0.50 ± 0	0.51 ±0.08	0.81 ± 0.2	0.4 ± 0.3
Sex	23 M/29F	10 M/19F	48 M/31F	25 M/15F	29 M/18F	135 M/112F

each element of the matrix was normalized by the total number of fibers detected per brain. Finally, we used the connectivity matrices to define each participant's brain network – as a set of nodes (ROIs) and edges (fiber pathways).

2.5   DWI-Derived Metrics

Graph theory: Structural networks are usually modeled as weighted or unweighted undirected graphs, containing a set of nodes, N, and edges, E. Using the weighted and binary form of the connectivity matrices, we computed some of most commonly cited graph theory metrics. The *nodal degree* describes the total number of edges that connect to a node, i: $k_i = \sum_{j \in N} a_{ij}$, where is the a_{ij} is a connections status between nodes i and j ($a_{ij} = 1$ if nodes i and j are connected and 0 otherwise); we assessed this at both the nodal (at each of the 68 ROIs) and global levels (average across all 68 ROIs). The weighted version of the nodal degree is also called the *nodal strength*, which we also included in our analysis. Nodal degree and strength have previously been found to be abnormal in patients with Alzheimer's disease, indicating a lower number of detectable fibers passing through a pair of ROIs [6, 7].

We also assessed the *characteristic path length* – a measure of network integration. This is computed as the total number of edges that need to be traversed to travel from one node to the other: $L = \frac{1}{n} \sum_{i \in N} L_i = \frac{1}{n} \frac{\sum_{j \in N, j \neq i} d_{ij}}{n-1}$. Here, N is the set of all nodes in the network. Presumably, shorter path lengths may be advantageous for more efficient information transfer, along with high levels of clustering [13]. This leads us to the next measures – *efficiency*, computed as the inverse of the average path length: $F = \sum_{i \in N} \frac{\sum_{j \in N, j \neq i} d_{ij}^{-1}}{n-1}$ and *clustering coefficient*: $CC_i = \sum_{i \in N} \frac{\frac{1}{2} \sum_{j,h \in N} a_{ij} a_{ih} a_{jh}}{k_i(k_i-1)}$.

Another frequently computed network measure is *modularity* – a statistical evaluation of the degree to which the network may be subdivided to separate groups of nodes, $Q = \sum_{u \in M} \left(F_{uu} - \left(\sum_{v \in M} F_{uv} \right)^2 \right)$; here, M is a non-overlapping module that the network is subdivided into, and F_{uv} is the proportion of links that connects nodes in module u to nodes in modules v [14].

Less frequently computed measures that we included are the network *flow coefficient*, defined as the number of edges of length 2 that link neighbors of a central node that pass through the node, divided by the total number of all possible edges [15]. Moreover, network *density* is defined as the ratio of detected connections to all possible connections [13]. Finally, *edge betweenness* is the fraction of all shortest edges in the network that contain a given edge [16].

Spectral graph theory: We computed our spectral features based on four Laplacians, which correspond to different transformations of the connectivity matrices. Our earlier work [17] found that different random walks on networks can offer different and complementary views of their structure. Here, we used four random walk Laplacians to capture informative structural features. The first is (1) the standard normalized Laplacian, which corresponds to the unbiased random walk with uniform time delays. It is defined as $L_{Norm}(G) = (D(G) - A(G))D(G)^{-1}$, where $A(G)$ is the adjacency matrix and $D(G)^{-1}$ is a delay factor inversely proportional to nodal degree. The second one is (2) the standard un-normalized Laplacian $L_{U-Norm}(G) = (D(G) - A(G))$, where $D(G)$ is the diagonal degree matrix. Furthermore, to capture the internal structure of each ROI, we assume that the random walk is delayed at each node. The delay was set to be proportional to each node's (3) gray matter volume, leading to the scaled Laplacian $L_V(G) = (D(G) - A(G))D(G)^{-1}T(G)^{-1}$ where $T(G)$ is the diagonal delay matrix and $T_{uu} = c_0 \cdot V_{graymatter_u}$. We also computed this using (4) gray matter thickness as the delay factor. The constant c_0 is chosen such that the trace of L_V is equal to that of L_{Norm}, so their spectra are properly normalized and comparable.

For the spectral features of each Laplacian, we calculated their top 12 eigenvalues as well as the total generalized volume. The number 12 is based on the community structure observed in each participant's network to reveal global organizational properties. In addition, we also used two spectral features based on the top 12 eigenvalues which may be useful for understanding network topology. One of them counts the number of 0 eigenvalues, and this indicates the number of disconnected components (ROIs) in the graph; the second is the sum of the eigenvalues describing the overall strength of community structures. Overall, these spectral graph theory measures describe levels of white matter connectedness between cortical areas of the brain.

2.6 Correlation Explanation (CorEx) for High-Dimensional Data

The newly developed method, CorEx, was used to identify the hierarchical structure in >700 widely used metrics extracted from DWIs and anatomical images, including the measures we have described already. CorEx goes beyond the study of pairwise, linear correlations by providing a principled information-theoretic method to decompose multivariate dependencies in high-dimensional data (http://www.github.com/gregversteeg/CorEx).

Let $X = (X1, \dots Xn)$ denote random variables in an arbitrary domain (Fig. 1). These could represent different experimental modalities or heterogeneous data types.

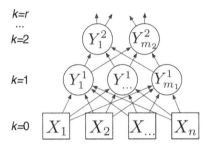

Fig. 1. The bottom row of variables (X_i's) represents measured quantities. Variables in higher layers are learned latent factors that explain the correlations in the layer beneath.

We assume that an observation is drawn from some unknown joint distribution $p_x(X = x)$, abbreviated p_x. We measure the relationships among the variables by a multivariate mutual information measure historically called "total correlation" (TC), although in modern terms it would be better described as measure of total dependence. TC is defined as:

$$TC(X) = D_{KL}\left(p(x) \middle\| \prod_i p(x_i)\right) = \sum_i H(X_i) - H(X)$$

Here, H denotes the Shannon entropy and D_{KL} is the Kullback-Leibler divergence. This quantity can be interpreted as the distance between the true data distribution and the expected distribution if all the variables were independent. This distance is zero if and only if the observed variables actually are independent. The total correlation among a group of variables, X, after conditioning on some other variable, Y, can be defined in terms of standard conditional entropies as $TC(X|Y) = \sum_i H(X_i|Y) - H(X|Y)$. We can measure the extent to which Y "explains" the correlations in X by looking at how much the total correlation is reduced after conditioning on Y:

$$TC(X;Y) = TC(X) - TC(X|Y) = \sum_i I(X_i;Y) - I(X;Y)$$

Here, $TC(X|Y)$ is zero and $TC(X;Y)$ maximized if and only if the distribution of X's conditioned on Y factorizes. This is the case if Y includes information about all the common causes of the X_i's (in which case we say that Y explains all the correlations in X).

The principle behind CorEx is to search for latent factors, $Y1, \ldots, Ym$, that maximize $TC(X;Y)$: $\max_{\forall j, p(y_j|x)} TC(X;Y)$. This optimization searches over all functions of x for the m representatives (shown as circular nodes in the middle row of Fig. 1) that are most informative about the data. Directly optimizing this objective is intractable for large m, so we optimize a lower bound $TC_L(X;Y)$ with two useful properties. First, we are able to optimize this lower bound efficiently (linear in the number of variables). Second, if we construct a hierarchy of representations in which Y^1 explains correlations in X, and Y^2 explains correlations in Y^1, etc., then to bound the information in X, we just add the contribution from each layer: $TC(X) \geq TC_L(X; Y^1) + TC_L(Y^1; Y^2) + \cdots$. For a more detailed discussion of bounds and optimization procedure, please refer to [3, 4].

The concrete result of this optimization is that each factor, Yi, is some learned function of the inputs that depends on some subset of the input variables. This dependence structure can be used to visualize hierarchical clusters. Also, since each Y_i is a (nonlinear) function of the inputs, we can check whether this new factor has any predictive value.

2.7 Significance of Each CorEx Variable for Predicting Cognitive Decline

Because latent factors learned by CorEx are optimized to capture common information among several variables, these factors are robust to noise in the observations. To determine if any of these factors were also predictive of cognitive decline (as measured by MMSE, ADAS-Cog and CDR-SOB scores separately), we ran a random effects regression in all 247 participants across the probabilities associated with each latent factor; we co-varied for age, sex, brain volume and diagnostic group and used scanning site as a random effects variable. We corrected for multiple comparison testing using the False Discovery Rate (FDR) ($q < 0.05$).

3 Results

Figure 2 shows a tree graph for the hierarchical structure of the top 100 latent factors for the neuroimaging derived measures in predicting cognitive decline. Measures are labeled with text, color-coded based on the measurement type, as indicated in the key. Other nodes in the graph represent latent factors discovered by CorEx, with factors at the first level of the hierarchy ($k = 1$ in Fig. 1) labeled with numbers 0...19. Links reflect learned functional relationships between variables and the thickness of an edge reflects the mutual information. The size of a latent factor node is based on the amount of multivariate mutual information among its children nodes. As expected, CorEx grouped measures within each category (gray matter, graph theory, spectral graph theory and white matter ROIs) more closely together and found strong correlations among them (thicker edge width indicates stronger correlation). Within each group of variables, latent factors 6, 7, 9, 14, 16 and 18 were associated with decline in MMSE scores (FDR critical $P = 0.014$); latent factors 6, 7, 9, 11, 14, 16 and 18 were associated with decline in ADAS-Cog scores (FDR critical $P = 9.0 \times 10^{-3}$) and finally, latent factors 7, 9, 11, 14 and 18 were associated with decline in CDR-SOB scores (FDR critical $P = 7.1 \times 10^{-3}$).

Gray matter thickness measures (latent factor groups 7 and 14) were the best predictors of cognitive decline (most significant/smallest observed p-values) across all imaging derived metrics. These most predictive and highly correlated measures were among areas known to be prevalent to Alzheimer's disease, such as the bilateral precuneus, entorhinal, inferior parietal and temporal lobes. The next most predictive measures of cognitive decline were gray matter volume (latent factor group 9), followed by graph theory nodal measures strength and nodal degree (latent factor groups 18 and 11). A set of eigenvalues from spectral graph theory, computed on the binary Laplacian matrices, were next most indicative of cognitive decline (latent factor group 16); these measures are sensitive to detecting network interconnectedness alterations in the connectome. Finally, gray matter surface area measures were least predictive of cognitive decline (latent factor group 6).

The group of white matter ROIs, described as functions of standard DTI metrics FA, MD, RD and AD, formed biologically meaningful patterns as discovered by CorEx. However, these measures were not significantly associated with cognitive decline.

4 Discussion

In this work, we show how a novel information-theoretic machine learning technique, CorEx, can reveal relationships among a diverse set of diffusion and anatomical derived measures from neuroimaging data. Measures of gray matter thickness were best predictors of cognitive decline, followed by gray matter volume, graph theory measures (strength and degree), spectral graph theory metrics and finally, gray matter surface area. We found that each structure discovered by CorEx is biologically meaningful and corresponds to anatomical and functional subdivisions in the brain, while the strongest correlations, also associated with cognitive decline, were among regions of the brain know to be prevalent to disease [6, 7, 18].

The hierarchical representation in Fig. 2 reveals several key observations about the data structure. First, as expected – the unsupervised algorithm identified highly correlated clusters among variables of the same type. Second, it determined that all neuroimaging-derived measures were correlated, although to a lesser extent than seen for the within group correlations. For instance, measures of gray matter thickness were clustered together with brain connectivity measures of strength and nodal degree. This might indicate that cortical thickness and white matter connectivity metrics contain shared information on the cognitive decline seen in Alzheimer's disease patients. Furthermore, spectral graph theory measures, also known as algebraic graph theory measures, were clustered with graph theory measures. This is expected as both groups of measures were computed using weighted or binary forms of the connectivity matrices. Spectral graph theory measures are less frequently applied in the context of disease, however, they were recently used to study connectivity patterns in Alzheimer's disease [1, 2] and found to be indicative of white matter breakdown in patients.

The most correlated measures associated with cognitive decline pointed to areas of the brain previously shown to atrophy in Alzheimer's disease [6, 7]. For instance, regions of interest such as the entorhinal, precuneus and areas of the temporal and parietal lobe were major components in the construction of latent factors significantly associated with decline of MMSE, ADAS-Cog and CDR-SOB scores. It is important to note that CorEx is based on model-free mathematical principles [3, 4] and determined these associations with no prior knowledge about the relationship between the anatomical and diffusion metrics. Overall, these measures were highly correlated making our system highly dimensional – implying that some common causes are responsible for generating these hierarchically represented correlations [3].

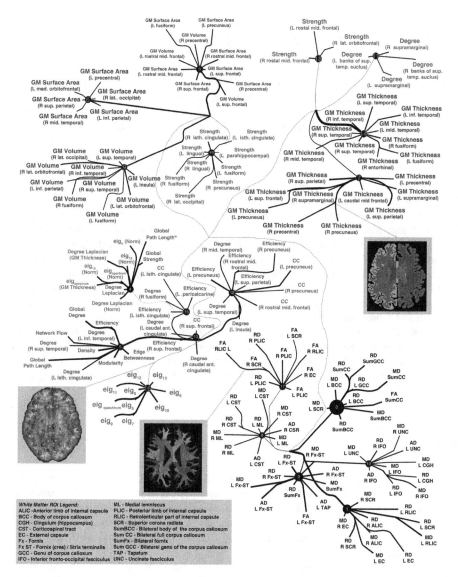

Fig. 2. Graph of latent factors for neuroimaging measures constructed by CorEx. Colors denote variable types (*purple* = gray matter (GM) thickness, volume and surface area; *blue* = graph theory measures; *red* = spectral graph theory measures; *black* = white matter ROI measures). Numbers in red mark latent factors that were significantly associated with cognitive decline; *eig = eigenvalue; Norm = normalized; CC = clustering coefficient; L = left hemisphere; R = right hemisphere.* (Color figure online)

The relationship between cortical atrophy and white matter connectivity breakdown is not well understood, yet it is critically important. Methods like CorEx, designed to identify groups of measures with high multivariate mutual information, might take us a few steps further in discovering the most descriptive metrics of neurodegenerative breakdown in the aging and diseased human brain.

Acknowledgments. Algorithm development and image analysis for this study was funded, in part, by grants to PT from the NIBIB (R01 EB008281, R01 EB008432) and by the NIA, NIBIB, NIMH, the National Library of Medicine, and the National Center for Research Resources (AG016570, AG040060, EB01651, MH097268, LM05639, RR019771 to PT). Data collection and sharing for this project was funded by ADNI (NIH Grant U01 AG024904). ADNI is funded by the National Institute on Aging, the National Institute of Biomedical Imaging and Bioengineering, and through contributions from the following: Abbott; Alzheimer's Association; Alzheimer's Drug Discovery Foundation; Amorfix Life Sciences Ltd.; AstraZeneca; Bayer HealthCare; BioClinica, Inc.; Biogen Idec Inc.; Bristol-Myers Squibb Company; Eisai Inc.; Elan Pharmaceuticals Inc.; Eli Lilly and Company; F. Hoffmann-La Roche Ltd and its affiliated company Genentech, Inc.; GE Healthcare; Innogenetics, N.V.; IXICO Ltd.; Janssen Alzheimer Immunotherapy Research & Development, LLC.; Johnson & Johnson Pharmaceutical Research & Development LLC.; Medpace, Inc.; Merck & Co., Inc.; Meso Scale Diagnostics, LLC.; Novartis Pharmaceuticals Corporation; Pfizer Inc.; Servier; Synarc Inc.; and Takeda Pharmaceutical Company. The Canadian Institutes of Health Research is providing funds to support ADNI clinical sites in Canada. Private sector contributions are facilitated by the Foundation for the National Institutes of Health. The grantee organization is the Northern California Institute for Research and Education, and the study is coordinated by the Alzheimer's Disease Cooperative Study at the University of California, San Diego. ADNI data are disseminated by the Laboratory for Neuro Imaging at the University of Southern California. This research was also supported by NIH grants P30 AG010129 and K01 AG030514 from the National Institute of General Medical Sciences; and by a Consortium grant (U54 EB020403) from the NIH Institutes contributing to the Big Data to Knowledge (BD2 K) Initiative, including the NIBIB and NCI.

References

1. Daianu, M., Jahanshad, N., Nir, T.M., Leonardo, C.D., Clifford, J.R.J., Weiner, M.W., Bernstein, M.A., Thompson, P.M.: Algebraic connectivity of brain networks shows patterns of segregation leading to reduced network robustness in Alzheimer's disease. In: O'Donnell, L., Nedjati-Gilani, G., Rathi, Y., Reisert, M., Schneider, T. (eds.) Medical Image Computing and Computer Assisted Intervention (MICCAI), Computational Diffusion MRI, pp. 55–64. Springer, Switzerland (2014)
2. Daianu, M., Mezher, A., Jahanshad, N., Hibar, D.P., Nir, T.M., Jack, C.R., Weiner, M.W., Bernstein, M.A., Thompson, P.M.: Spectral graph theory and graph energy metrics show evidence for the Alzheimer's disease disconnection syndrome in APOE-4 gene carriers. In: IEEE International Symposium of Biomedical Imaging (ISBI), pp. 458–461 (2015)
3. Ver Steeg, G., Galstyan, A.: Maximally informative hierarchical representations of high-dimensional data. In: Artificial Intelligence and Statistics Conference (2014)
4. Ver Steeg, G., Galstyan, A.: Discovering structure in high-dimensional data through correlation explanation. In: Advances in Neural Information Processing Systems (2014)

5. Madsen, S.K., Ver Steeg, G., Daianu, M., Mezher, A., Jahanshad, N., Nir, T.M., Hua, X., Gutman, B.A., Galstyan, A., Thompson, P.M.: Relative value of diverse brain MRI and blood-based biomarkers for predicting cognitive decline in the elderly. In: The International Society for Optics and Photonics (SPIE), Medical Imaging 2016: Image Processing (2015, in Press)
6. Daianu, M., Jahanshad, N., Nir, T.M., Jack Jr., C.R., Weiner, M.W., Bernstein, M.A., Thompson, P.M., Alzheimer's Disease Neuroimaging, I.: Rich club analysis in the Alzheimer's disease connectome reveals a relatively undisturbed structural core network. Hum. Brain Mapp. **36**, 3087–3103 (2015)
7. Daianu, M., Jahanshad, N., Nir, T.M., Toga, A.W., Jack Jr., C.R., Weine, M.W., Thompson, P.M., Alzheimer's Disease Neuroimaging, I.: Breakdown of brain connectivity between normal aging and Alzheimer's disease: a structural k-core network analysis. Brain Connectivity **3**, 407–422 (2013)
8. Daianu, M., Dennis, E.L., Jahanshad, N., Nir, T.M., Toga, A.W., Jack, C.R., Weiner, M.W., Thompson, P.M.: Alzheimer's disease disrupts rich club organization in brain connectivity networks. In: IEEE International Symposium of Biomedical Imaging (ISBI), pp. 266–269 (2013)
9. Mori, S., Oishi, K., Jiang, H., Jiang, L., Li, X., Akhter, K., Hua, K., Faria, A.V., Mahmood, A., Woods, R., Toga, A.W., Pike, G.B., Neto, P.R., Evans, A., Zhang, J., Huang, H., Miller, M.I., van Zijl, P., Mazziotta, J.: Stereotaxic white matter atlas based on diffusion tensor imaging in an ICBM template. NeuroImage **40**, 570–582 (2008)
10. Leow, A., Huang, S.-C., Geng, A., Becker, J., Davis, S., Toga, A.W., Thompson, P.: Inverse consistent mapping in 3D deformable image registration: its construction and statistical properties. In: Christensen, G.E., Sonka, M. (eds.) IPMI 2005. LNCS, vol. 3565, pp. 493–503. Springer, Heidelberg (2005)
11. Fischl, B.: Automatically parcellating the human cerebral cortex. Cereb. Cortex **14**, 11–22 (2004)
12. Desikan, R.S., Segonne, F., Fischl, B., Quinn, B.T., Dickerson, B.C., Blacker, D., Buckner, R.L., Dale, A.M., Maguire, R.P., Hyman, B.T., Albert, M.S., Killiany, R.J.: An automated labeling system for subdividing the human cerebral cortex on MRI scans into gyral based regions of interest. NeuroImage **31**, 968–980 (2006)
13. Sporns, O.: The human connectome: a complex network. Ann. N. Y. Acad. Sci. **1224**, 109–125 (2011)
14. Rubinov, M., Sporns, O.: Complex network measures of brain connectivity: uses and interpretations. NeuroImage **52**, 1059–1069 (2010)
15. Honey, C.J., Kotter, R., Breakspear, M., Sporns, O.: Network structure of cerebral cortex shapes functional connectivity on multiple time scales. Proc. Natl. Acad. Sci. U.S.A. **104**, 10240–10245 (2007)
16. Brandes, U.: A faster algorithm for betweenness centrality. J. Math. Sociol. **25**, 163–177 (2001)
17. Ghosh, R., Lerman, K., Teng, S.H., Yan, X.: The interplay between dynamics and networks: centrality, communities, and cheeger inequality. Soc. Inf. Netw. (2014)
18. Roussotte, F.F., Daianu, M., Jahanshad, N., Leonardo, C.D., Thompson, P.M.: Neuroimaging and genetic risk for Alzheimer's disease and addiction-related degenerative brain disorders. Brain Imaging Behav. **8**, 217–233 (2014)

Relationship Induced Multi-atlas Learning for Alzheimer's Disease Diagnosis

Mingxia Liu[1,2], Daoqiang Zhang[2], Ehsan Adeli-Mosabbeb[1],
and Dinggang Shen[1(✉)]

[1] Department of Radiology and BRIC, University of North Carolina at Chapel Hill,
Chapel Hill, NC 27599, USA
dgshen@med.unc.edu
[2] School of Computer Science and Technology,
Nanjing University of Aeronautics and Astronautics, Nanjing 210016, China

Abstract. Multi-atlas based methods using magnetic resonance imaging (MRI) have been recently proposed for automatic diagnosis of Alzheimer's disease (AD) and its prodromal stage, i.e., mild cognitive impairment (MCI). However, most existing multi-atlas based methods simply average or concatenate features generated from multiple atlases, which ignores the important underlying structure information of multi-atlas data. In this paper, we propose a novel relationship induced multi-atlas learning (RIML) method for AD/MCI classification. Specifically, we first register each brain image onto multiple selected atlases separately, through which multiple sets of feature representations can be extracted. To exploit the structure information of data, we develop a relationship induced sparse feature selection method, by employing two regularization terms to model the relationships among atlases and among subjects. Finally, we learn a classifier based on selected features in each atlas space, followed by an ensemble classification strategy to combine multiple classifiers for making a final decision. Experimental results on the Alzheimer's Disease Neuroimaging Initiative (ADNI) database demonstrate that our method achieves significant performance improvement for AD/MCI classification, compared with several state-of-the-art methods.

1 Introduction

Brain morphometric pattern analysis using magnetic resonance imaging (MRI) is one of the most popular approaches for automatic diagnosis of Alzheimer's disease (AD) and its early stage, i.e., mild cognitive impairment (MCI). In these methods, all subjects are spatially normalized onto a common space (i.e., a predefined atlas), through which the same brain region across different subjects can be compared [1]. However, due to the potential bias associated with the use of a specific atlas, feature representations extracted from a single atlas may not be sufficient to reveal the underlying complicated differences between populations of disease-affected patients and normal controls (NC).

Recently, several studies [2–4] have shown that multi-atlas based methods usually achieve more accurate diagnosis results than single-atlas based ones.

© Springer International Publishing Switzerland 2016
B. Menze et al. (Eds.): MCV Workshop 2015, LNCS 9601, pp. 24–33, 2016.
DOI: 10.1007/978-3-319-42016-5_3

In multi-atlas based methods, one brain image is non-linearly registered onto multiple atlases, and thus multiple feature representations can be generated for this image. Using multiple atlases could reduce errors due to misregistration, which is helpful for improving subsequent learning performance. However, most of existing multi-atlas based methods simply average or concatenate multiple sets of features generated from multiple atlases, which do not take advantage of the underlying structure information [5,6] of multi-atlas data. In fact, there exists some important structure information, e.g., the relationships among atlases and among subjects. Intuitively, modeling such relationships can bring more prior information into the learning process, which can further boost the learning performance. However, to the best of our knowledge, previous multi-atlas based methods seldome utilize such relationship information in their models.

In this paper, we propose a relationship induced multi-atlas learning (RIML) method for AD/MCI classification. We first non-linearly register each brain image onto multiple selected atlases, and then extract multiple sets of feature representations for each subject from those atlas spaces. Next, we develop a novel relationship induced sparse feature selection model, by considering the relationships among multiple atlases and among different subjects. Finally, we develop an ensemble classification method to better make use of feature representations generated from multiple atlases. Experimental results on the ADNI database demonstrate the efficacy of our method.

2   Proposed Method

Figure 1 illustrates the overview of our proposed method, which includes three major steps: (1) feature extraction, (2) relationship induced sparse feature selection, and (3) ensemble classification. In the first step, brain images are non-linearly registered onto multiple selected atlases separately, and then multiple sets of volumetric features are extracted for each subject in each atlas space. Afterwards, our proposed relationship induced sparse feature selection method is used to select the most discriminative features by considering the underlying structure information in multi-atlas data. Finally, multiple SVM classifiers are constructed based on multiple sets of selected features, followed by an ensemble classification strategy to combine the outputs of multiple classifiers.

2.1   Feature Extraction

For all studied subjects, we first perform a standard pre-processing procedure on the T1-weighted MR brain images. Specifically, we first use the non-parametric non-uniform bias correction [7] method to correct intensity in-homogeneity. Next, we perform skull stripping [8], and double check it to ensure the clean removal of skull and dura. Then, we remove the cerebellum by warping a labeled atlas to each skull-stripped image. Afterwards, we apply the FAST method [9] to segment each brain image into three tissues: gray matter (GM), white matter (WM), and cerebrospinal fluid (CSF). Here, we only use the GM density map

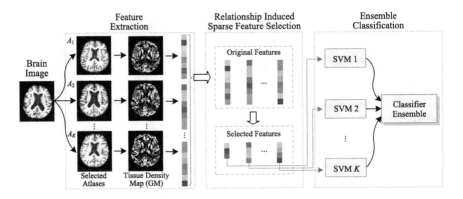

Fig. 1. The overview of our proposed RIML method.

in our feature set, because GM is mostly affected by AD and is widely used in the literature [3,10]. Finally, all brain images are affine-aligned by FLIRT [11].

To obtain multiple atlases, we adopt the affinity propagation (AP) clustering algorithm [12] to partition the whole population of AD and NC images into K non-overlapping groups. The exemplar image of each group is then selected as an atlas, and a total of $K = 10$ atlases (i.e., $A_1, \cdots, A_{10}$) are obtained (see Fig. 2) empirically in this study. We then employ these atlases to capture multiple sets of feature representations for each subject by performing feature extraction as described in [10]. Specifically, for a given subject with three segmented tissues (i.e., GM, WM and CSF), its brain image is first non-linearly registered onto K atlases separately by using a high-dimensional elastic warping tool, i.e., HAM-MER [13]. Then, based on these K estimated deformation fields, for each tissue we quantify its voxel-wise tissue density map [14] in each of K atlas spaces, to reflect the unique deformation behavior of a given subject with respect to each specific atlas. In this study, we only use the gray matter (GM) density map for feature extraction and classification, since GM is mostly affected by AD and is widely used in the literature [4,15]. After registration and quantification, we group voxel-wise morphometric features into regional features by using the clustering method proposed in [10] for adaptive feature grouping, followed by a Watershed segmentation [16] process for obtaining the region of interest (ROI) partitions for each of multiple atlases. Here, each atlas will yield its unique ROI partition, because different tissue density maps of the same subject are generated from different atlases. To improve the discriminative power as well as the robustness of volumetric features computed from each ROI, we further refine ROI by choosing the voxels with reasonable representation power. To be specific, we first select the most relevant voxel according to the Pearson correlation between this voxels tissue density values and class labels among all training subjects. Then, we iteratively include the neighboring voxels until no increase in Pearson correlation when adding new voxels. Such voxel selection process will lead to a voxel set for a specific region, and then the mean of tissue density values of those selected voxels can be computed as the feature representation for this region. Such voxel selection process is important in helping eliminate irrelevant and noisy features, confirmed by several previous studies [4,15,17]. Finally, the top 1500 most discriminative ROI features are selected in each atlas space in this study. By using K atlases, one subject is represented by K sets of feature vectors, where each feature vector is of 1500 dimensions.

A_1 A_2 A_3 A_4 A_5 A_6 A_7 A_8 A_9 A_{10}

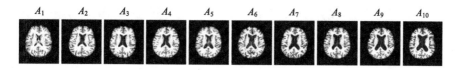

Fig. 2. Selected atlases achieved by the AP clustering algorithm.

2.2   Relationship Induced Sparse Feature Selection

Since multiple atlases are used in this study, feature representations for each subject are high-dimensional, while the number of subjects is usually very limited. In such a case, features could be noisy or redundant, which could degrate the performances of subsequent classifiers [5,18–20]. To this end, we propose a relationship induced sparse feature selection algorithm to find the most informative features in multi-atlas data. Assume we have K learning tasks (corresponding to K atlases). Denote $\mathbf{X}^k = [\mathbf{x}_1^k, \mathbf{x}_2^k, \cdots, \mathbf{x}_n^k, \cdots, \mathbf{x}_N^k]^\top \in \mathbb{R}^{N \times D}$ as the training data for the kth learning task with N training subjects, where $\mathbf{x}_n^k$ represents the column feature vector for the nth training subject in the kth atlas space. Let $\mathbf{y} = [y_1, y_2, \cdots, y_n, \cdots, y_N]^\top \in \mathbb{R}^N$ represent the column response vector for the training data, where $y_n \in \{-1, 1\}$ is the class label for the nth subject. Denote $\mathbf{W} = [\mathbf{w}^1, \mathbf{w}^2, \cdots, \mathbf{w}^k, \cdots, \mathbf{w}^K] \in \mathbb{R}^{D \times K}$ as the weight matrix for K tasks, where $\mathbf{w}^k \in \mathbb{R}^D$ is a column weight vector for the kth task, and $\mathbf{w}_d \in \mathbb{R}^K$ that will be used below as the dth row of $\mathbf{W}$. To encourage the sparsity of $\mathbf{W}$, and to select the most informative features in each atlas space, we propose the following multi-task sparse feature learning model:

$$\min_{\mathbf{W}} \sum_{k=1}^{K} \|\mathbf{y} - \mathbf{X}^k \mathbf{w}^k\|^2 + \lambda_1 \|\mathbf{W}\|_{1,1} \tag{1}$$

where the first term is the empirical loss on the training data, and $\|\mathbf{W}\|_{1,1} = \sum_{d=1}^{D} |\mathbf{w}_d|$ is the sum of ℓ_1-norm of the rows of $\mathbf{W}$ to ensure that only a small subset of features will be selected in each task.

In (1), a linear mapping function (i.e., $f(\mathbf{x}) = \mathbf{x}^\top \mathbf{w}$) is learned to transform the data in original feature space to a one-dimensional label space, which only considers the relationship between samples and class labels. Nevertheless, there exists some other important structure information when we use multiple atlases for extracting feature representations, e.g., (1) the relationship among multiple atlases, and (2) the relationship among subjects. As illustrated in the left panel of Fig. 3, one subject $\mathbf{x}_n$ is represented as $\mathbf{x}_n^{k_1}$ in the k_1^{th} atlas space, and as

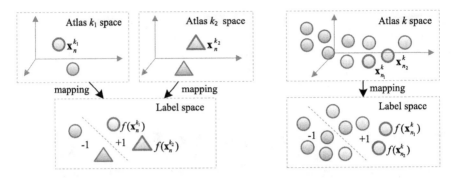

Fig. 3. Illustration of the relationship between two atlases (left panel), and the relationship between two subjects in the same atlas space (right panel).

$\mathbf{x}_n^{k_2}$ in the $k_2{}^{\text{th}}$ atlas space, respectively. After being mapped to the label space, they should be close to each other (i.e., $f(\mathbf{x}_n^{k_1})$ should be similar to $f(\mathbf{x}_n^{k_2})$), since they represent the same subject. Similarly, as shown in the right panel of Fig. 3, if two subjects $\mathbf{x}_{n_1}^k$ and $\mathbf{x}_{n_2}^k$ in the kth atlas space are very similar, their estimated label information should be also similar, i.e., the distance between $f(\mathbf{x}_{n_1}^k)$ and $f(\mathbf{x}_{n_2}^k)$ should be small. To achieve these goals, we first introduce a novel atlas-relationship induced regularization term P as follows:

$$P = \sum_{n=1}^{N} \sum_{k_1=1}^{K} \sum_{k_2=1}^{K} \left(f(\mathbf{x}_n^{k_1}) - f(\mathbf{x}_n^{k_2}) \right)^2 = \sum_{n=1}^{N} tr\left((\mathbf{B}_n \mathbf{W})^{\top} \mathbf{L}_n (\mathbf{B}_n \mathbf{W}) \right) \quad (2)$$

where $tr(\cdot)$ denotes the trace of a square matrix, $\mathbf{B}_n = [\mathbf{x}_n^1, \cdots, \mathbf{x}_n^K]^{\top} \in \mathbb{R}^{K \times D}$ represents the nth subject with multiple sets of features generated from K atlas spaces, and $\mathbf{L}_n \in \mathbb{R}^{K \times K}$ is a diagonal matrix with diagonal elements equal to $K - 1$ and all the other elements as -1. By using (2), we can model the relationships among multiple atlases explicitly.

We then also propose a subject-relationship induced regularizer Q as follows:

$$Q = \sum_{k=1}^{K} \sum_{n_1=1}^{N} \sum_{n_2=1}^{N} S_{n_1 n_2}^k \left(f(\mathbf{x}_{n_1}^k) - f(\mathbf{x}_{n_2}^k) \right)^2 = \sum_{k=1}^{K} \left(\mathbf{X}^k \mathbf{w}^k \right)^{\top} \mathbf{L}^k \left(\mathbf{X}^k \mathbf{w}^k \right) \quad (3)$$

where $\mathbf{X}^k$ denotes the data matrix in the kth learning task, and $S_{n_1 n_2}^k$ represents the similarity between the n_1^{th} subject and the n_2^{th} subject in the kth atlas space. Here, $S_{n_1 n_2}^k$ is defined as $e^{-\frac{\|\mathbf{x}_{n_1}^k - \mathbf{x}_{n_2}^k\|^2}{\sigma}}$ if $\mathbf{x}_{n_1}^k$ and $\mathbf{x}_{n_2}^k$ are neighbors, and 0 otherwise. Therefore, $\mathbf{S}^k = \{S_{n_1 n_2}^k\}_{n_1,n_2=1}^N \in \mathbb{R}^{N \times N}$ could be a similarity matrix with elements defining the similarities between subjects. Then, $\mathbf{L}^k = \mathbf{D}^k - \mathbf{S}^k$ represents the Laplacian matrix, where $\mathbf{D}^k$ is a diagonal matrix with the element $D_{n_1 n_1}^k = \sum_{n_2=1}^{N} S_{n_1 n_2}^k$. It is easy to see that (3) aims to preserve the local neighboring structure of original data during the mapping, through which the relationships among subjects can be captured explicitly.

By incorporating two relationship induced regularization terms defined in (2) and (3) into (1), our proposed relationship induced sparse feature selection model can be finally formulated as follows:

$$\min_{\mathbf{W}} \sum_{k=1}^{K} \|\mathbf{y} - \mathbf{X}^k \mathbf{w}^k\|^2 + \lambda_1 \|\mathbf{W}\|_{1,1} + \lambda_2 P + \lambda_3 Q \qquad (4)$$

where λ_1, λ_2 and λ_3 are positive constants to balance the relative contributions of those four terms in (4), and their values can be determined via inner cross-validation on training data. In (4), the second term is used to find the most discriminative features, and the last two terms are to capture the relationships among atlases and among subjects. Since the objective function in (4) is convex but non-smooth because of the non-smooth term $l_{1,1}$-norm, we adopt a smooth approximation algorithm [21] to solve the proposed problem.

2.3   Ensemble Classification

To better make use of feature representations generated from multiple atlases, we further propose using an ensemble classification approach. Particularly, after feature selection using our relationship induced sparse feature selection algorithm, we obtain K feature subsets from the K different atlases. Based on these selected features, we then construct K SVM classifiers separately, with each classifier corresponding to a specific atlas space. Next, we adopt the majority voting strategy, which is a simple and effective classifier fusion method, to combine the outputs of K SVM classifiers for making a final decision. In this way, the class label of a new test subject can be determined by majority voting for the outputs of those K classifiers.

3   Experiments

3.1   Subjects and Experimental Settings

We evaluate our method on T1-weighted MRI data in ADNI-1 for AD/MCI classification. In the experiments, there are totally 459 subjects randomly selected from those scanned with 1.5 T scanners, including 97 AD, 128 NC, 117 progressive MCI (pMCI), and 117 stable MCI (sMCI) subjects. We perform two groups of experiments, including AD vs. NC classification and pMCI vs. sMCI classification. We compare our RIML method with four widely used feature selection methods, including Pearson correlation (PC), COMPARE [10], t-test, and LASSO [22]. We first use single-atlas (sa) based methods to perform classification, denoted as PC_sa, COMPARE_sa, t-test_sa, and LASSO_sa. Then, we adopt two strategies to deal with features from multiple atlases, i.e., feature concatenation and ensemble. In feature concatenation methods (including PC_con, COMPARE_con, t-test_con, and LASSO_con), we first concatenate features extracted from K atlases ($K = 10$ in this study), and then use a specific feature selection method to select features, followed by a SVM classifier. In ensemble methods (including PC_ens, COMPARE_ens, t-test_ens, and LASSO_ens), we first select features in each atlas space by using a specific feature selection algorithm, and then construct K SVM classifiers, followed by an ensemble classification process (see Fig. 1).

In the experiments, we use a 10-fold cross-validation strategy to evaluate the performance of different methods, and record the average results among those 10 folds. The regularization parameters in (4) and that for LASSO are chosen from $\{10^{-10}, 10^{-9}, \cdots, 10^{0}\}$, and the p-value in t-test method is chosen from $\{0.05, 0.08, 0.10, 0.12, 0.15\}$ via inner cross-validation on the training data. We use the linear SVM with default parameters as classifier, and evaluate the performance of different methods via four criteria, including classification accuracy (ACC), sensitivity (SEN), specificity (SPE), and the area under the receiver operating characteristic curve (AUC).

3.2   Results and Analysis

First, we report the results achieved by four single-atlas based methods and nine multi-atlas based methods in Table 1. For the single-atlas based methods, the averaged results using K individual atlases are provided. From Table 1, we can observe three main points: First, multi-atlas based methods generally achieve better performances than single-atlas based methods (i.e., PC_sa, COMPARE_sa, t-test_sa, and LASSO_sa). For instance, in AD vs. NC classification, the best accuracy achieved by single-atlas based methods is only 84.32 % (by LASSO_sa), which is usually lower than those of multi-atlas based methods. Second, when using multiple atlases, our proposed ensemble strategy (i.e., PC_en, COMPARE_ens, t-test_ens, and LASSO_ens) usually outperforms their counterparts using feature concatenation strategy (i.e., PC_con, COMPARE_con, t-test_con, and LASSO_con). Third, in most cases, our RIML method achieves better results than the compared methods. Also, our method

Then, we compare the results achieved by RIML with several state-of-the-art multi-atlas based methods using MRI data from ADNI, with results shown in Table 2. From Table 2, it is obvious that our RIML method generally outperforms the other three methods in both AD vs. NC classification and pMCI vs. sMCI

Table 1. Comparison of RIML with different methods in two classification tasks.

Method		AD vs. NC				pMCI vs. sMCI			
		ACC (%)	SEN (%)	SPE (%)	AUC (%)	ACC (%)	SEN (%)	SPE (%)	AUC (%)
Single-atlas	PC_sa	84.00	79.53	87.45	76.92	68.49	67.80	69.10	62.85
	COMPARE_sa	84.18	75.33	89.17	78.70	70.06	68.08	72.02	63.56
	t-test_sa	76.27	68.50	83.01	74.96	61.99	64.93	73.11	65.16
	LASSO_sa	84.32	81.66	86.36	84.02	72.06	72.04	72.02	72.03
Multi-atlas	PC_con	84.01	81.56	89.23	81.91	72.78	74.62	70.91	72.45
	COMPARE_con	84.93	80.11	87.03	79.07	73.35	75.76	70.83	74.05
	t-test_con	81.87	70.77	**90.71**	81.78	61.60	64.32	75.01	71.63
	LASSO_con	86.62	84.78	89.80	87.29	71.49	76.06	66.67	71.36
	PC_ens	85.59	82.44	89.93	91.51	73.92	73.38	72.32	76.29
	COMPARE_ens	86.61	85.44	89.23	90.85	75.56	75.75	73.48	76.58
	t-test_ens	84.31	74.56	89.70	88.78	63.36	60.60	71.74	63.33
	LASSO_ens	87.27	84.78	89.23	92.79	75.32	81.36	69.17	76.02
	RIML(ours)	**93.06**	**94.85**	90.49	**95.79**	**79.25**	**87.92**	**75.54**	**83.44**

Table 2. Comparison with the state-of-the-art methods using MRI data of ADNI.

Method	AD vs. NC			pMCI vs. sMCI		
	ACC (%)	SEN (%)	SPE (%)	ACC (%)	SEN (%)	SPE (%)
Wolz et al. [2]	89.00	85.00	93.00	68.00	67.00	69.00
Koikkalainen et al. [3]	86.00	81.00	91.00	72.10	77.00	71.00
Min et al. [15]	91.64	88.56	**93.85**	72.41	72.12	72.58
RIML(ours)	**93.06**	**94.85**	90.49	**79.25**	**87.92**	**75.54**

classification. Although the study in [15] reported the best specificity in AD vs. NC classification, its accuracy and sensitivity are lower than those of the proposed RIML method.

3.3 Diversity Analysis

In order to understand how our ensemble classification method works, we further plot a diversity-error diagram [23] to evaluate the level of agreement between the outputs of two classifiers. In Fig. 4, we show diagrams achieved by five ensemble-based methods. For each method, the corresponding ensemble contains K ($K = 10$ in this study) individual SVM classifiers. In a diversity-error diagram, the value on the x-axis denotes the kappa diversity of a pair of classifiers in the ensemble, and that on the y-axis represents the averaged individual error of a pair of classifiers. The most desirable pairs of classifiers will be close to the bottom left corner of the diagram, since a small value of kappa diversity indicates better diversity and a small value of averaged error indicates a better accuracy. For visual evaluation of relative positions of kappa-error point clouds, we also plot the centroids of clouds for different methods in Fig. 4 (denoted as squares). It can be seen from Fig. 4 that our RIML method usually yields better diversity and lower classification error than the other four methods, implying that RIML can achieve a better trade-off between the classification error and the classifier

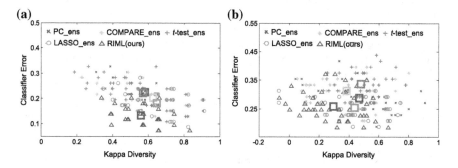

Fig. 4. Diversity-error diagrams of classifiers achieved by five ensemble-based methods in (a) AD vs. NC classification, and (b) pMCI vs. sMCI classification.

diversity than the compared methods. That is, it builds a classifier ensemble based on the reasonably diverse and accurate individual components.

4 Conclusion

In this paper, we have proposed a relationship induced multi-atlas learning (RIML) method for AD/MCI classification. Specifically, we first extracted feature representations from multiple selected atlases, and then proposed a relationship induced sparse feature selection method, followed by an ensemble classification method. Experimental results on the ADNI database demonstrate that our RIML method achieves significant performance improvement in both AD vs. NC classification and pMCI vs. sMCI classification, compared with several state-of-the-art methods.

Acknowledgements. This study was supported by NIH grants (EB006733, EB008374, EB009634, MH100217, AG041721, and AG042599), the National Natural Science Foundation of China (Nos. 61422204, 61473149), the Jiangsu Natural Science Foundation for Distinguished Young Scholar (No. BK20130034), and the NUAA Fundamental Research Fund under grant number NE2013105.

References

1. Cuingnet, R., Gerardin, E., Tessieras, J., Auzias, G., Lehéricy, S., Habert, M.O., Chupin, M., Benali, H., Colliot, O., Initiative, A.D.N.: Automatic classification of patients with Alzheimer's disease from structural MRI: a comparison of ten methods using the ADNI database. NeuroImage **56**(2), 766–781 (2011)
2. Wolz, R., Julkunen, V., Koikkalainen, J., Niskanen, E., Zhang, D.P., Rueckert, D., Soininen, H., Lötjönen, J., Alzheimer's Disease Neuroimaging Initiative: Multi-method analysis of MRI images in early diagnostics of Alzheimer's disease. PLOS ONE **6**(10), e25446 (2011)
3. Koikkalainen, J., Lötjönen, J., Thurfjell, L., Rueckert, D., Waldemar, G., Soininen, H., Alzheimer's Disease Neuroimaging Initiative: Multi-template tensor-based morphometry: application to analysis of Alzheimer's disease. NeuroImage **56**(3), 1134–1144 (2011)
4. Liu, M., Zhang, D., Shen, D.: View-centralized multi-atlas classification for Alzheimer's disease diagnosis. Hum. Brain Mapp. **36**, 1847–1865 (2015)
5. Liu, M., Zhang, D.: Pairwise constraint-guided sparse learning for feature selection. IEEE Transactions on Cybernetics **46**, 298–310 (2015)
6. Liu, M., Zhang, D., Chen, S., Xue, H.: Joint binary classifier learning for ECOC-based multi-class classification. IEEE Trans. Pattern Anal. Mach. Intell. (2015)
7. Sled, J.G., Zijdenbos, A.P., Evans, A.C.: A nonparametric method for automatic correction of intensity nonuniformity in MRI data. IEEE Trans. Med. Imaging **17**(1), 87–97 (1998)
8. Wang, Y., Nie, J., Yap, P.T., Li, G., Shi, F., Geng, X., Guo, L., Shen, D., Initiative, A.D.N.: Knowledge-guided robust MRI brain extraction for diverse large-scale neuroimaging studies on humans and non-human primates. PLOS ONE **9**(1), e77810 (2014)

9. Zhang, Y., Brady, M., Smith, S.: Segmentation of brain MR images through a hidden Markov random field model and the expectation-maximization algorithm. IEEE Trans. Med. Imaging **20**(1), 45–57 (2001)
10. Fan, Y., Shen, D., Gur, R.C., Gur, R.E., Davatzikos, C.: COMPARE: classification of morphological patterns using adaptive regional elements. IEEE Trans. Med. Imaging **26**(1), 93–105 (2007)
11. Jenkinson, M., Smith, S.: A global optimisation method for robust affine registration of brain images. Med. Image Anal. **5**(2), 143–156 (2001)
12. Frey, B.J., Dueck, D.: Clustering by passing messages between data points. Science **315**(5814), 972–976 (2007)
13. Shen, D., Davatzikos, C.: Hammer: hierarchical attribute matching mechanism for elastic registration. IEEE Trans. Med. Imaging **21**(11), 1421–1439 (2002)
14. Goldszal, A.F., Davatzikos, C., Pham, D.L., Yan, M.X., Bryan, R.N., Resnick, S.M.: An image-processing system for qualitative and quantitative volumetric analysis of brain images. J. Comput. Assist. Tomogr. **22**(5), 827–837 (1998)
15. Min, R., Wu, G., Cheng, J., Wang, Q., Shen, D.: Multi-atlas based representations for Alzheimer's disease diagnosis. Hum. Brain Mapp. **35**(10), 5052–5070 (2014)
16. Vincent, L., Soille, P.: Watersheds in digital spaces: an efficient algorithm based on immersion simulations. IEEE Trans. Pattern Anal. Mach. Intell. **6**, 583–598 (1991)
17. Jin, Y., Shi, Y., Zhan, L., Gutman, B.A., de Zubicaray, G.I., McMahon, K.L., Wright, M.J., Toga, A.W., Thompson, P.M.: Automatic clustering of white matter fibers in brain diffusion mri with an application to genetics. Neuroimage **100**, 75–90 (2014)
18. Gao, Y., Wang, M., Tao, D., Ji, R., Dai, Q.: 3-d object retrieval and recognition with hypergraph analysis. IEEE Trans. Image Process. **21**(9), 4290–4303 (2012)
19. Ji, R., Gao, Y., Hong, R., Liu, Q., Tao, D., Li, X.: Spectral-spatial constraint hyperspectral image classification. IEEE Trans. Geosci. Remote Sens. **52**(3), 1811–1824 (2014)
20. Liu, M., Miao, L., Zhang, D.: Two-stage cost-sensitive learning for software defect prediction. IEEE Trans. Reliab. **63**(2), 676–686 (2014)
21. Nesterov, Y.: Smooth minimization of non-smooth functions. Math. Program. **103**(1), 127–152 (2005)
22. Tibshirani, R.: Regression shrinkage and selection via the lasso. J. R. Stat. Soc. Ser. B (Methodological) **58**, 267–288 (1996)
23. Rodriguez, J.J., Kuncheva, L.I., Alonso, C.J.: Rotation forest: a new classifier ensemble method. IEEE Trans. Pattern Anal. Mach. Intell. **28**(10), 1619–1630 (2006)

Atlas Exploitation and Avoidance

Hierarchical Multi-Organ Segmentation Without Registration in 3D Abdominal CT Images

Vasileios Zografos[1]([✉]), Alexander Valentinitsch[1,2], Markus Rempfler[1],
Federico Tombari[1,2], and Bjoern Menze[1]

[1] Computer Aided Medical Procedures and Augmented Reality,
TUM, Munich, Germany
vasileios@zografos.org
[2] Department of Diagnostic and Interventional Neuroradiology,
TUM, Munich, Germany

Abstract. We present a novel framework for the segmentation of multiple organs in 3D abdominal CT images, which does not require registration with an atlas. Instead we use discriminative classifiers that have been trained on an array of 3D volumetric features and implicitly model the appearance of the organs of interest. We fully leverage all the available data and extract the features from inside supervoxels at multiple levels of detail. Parallel to this, we employ a hierarchical auto-context classification scheme, where the trained classifier at each level is applied back onto the image to provide additional features for the next level. The final segmentation is obtained using a hierarchical conditional random field fusion step. We have tested our approach on 20 contrast enhanced CT images of 8 organs from the VISCERAL dataset and obtained results comparable to the state-of-the-art methods that require very costly registration steps and a much larger corpus of training data. Our method is accurate, fast and general enough that may be applied to a variety of realistic clinical applications and any number of organs.

1 Introduction

Multiple organ segmentation in abdominal computer tomography (CT) images can be an important step to computer aided diagnosis and computer assisted surgery. Existing work in automated multi-organ segmentation can be roughly divided into *registration based* and *classification based*. Registration methods include statistical shape models (SSM) [1], probabilistic atlases (PA) [2,3] and multi-altas techniques (MA) [4]. SSM approaches work by employing several shape or appearance models, usually in conjunction with hierarchical object localisation. Although SSM can produce accurate segmentations, they require good initialisation otherwise registration between the SSM the organs will fail. PA are more robust to registration with a target image since they incorporate global spatial information as well as inter-organ spatial relationships. However, both SSM and PA cannot handle large inter-subject variabilities, so research

© Springer International Publishing Switzerland 2016
B. Menze et al. (Eds.): MCV Workshop 2015, LNCS 9601, pp. 37–46, 2016.
DOI: 10.1007/978-3-319-42016-5_4

(a)

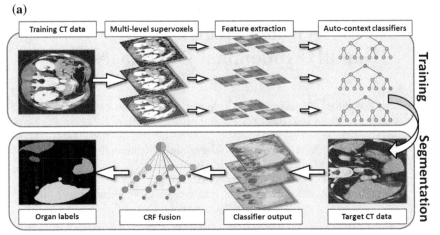

The main components in our registration-free CT segmentation approach.

(b)

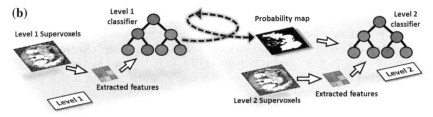

Hierarchical auto-context between two subsequent levels.

Fig. 1. Proposed method outline (a) and details of the hierarchical auto-context (b)

has moved on to target-specific MA solutions, which have shown to be superior to single model/atlas approaches. All registration-based methods are limited in that they require every organ to be present and to have stable locations between training and test images (localised spatial support). Furthermore, non-rigid registration can be very time consuming. Especially for MA approaches, it is necessary to have all the atlases available during segmentation time and register the target image with each atlas separately. The classification-based methods on the other hand, are not plagued by the same problems as registration-based approaches. Instead, they can predict the probability that a voxel belongs to a specific object based on previously seen data. Most classification-based methods [5,6] use some flavour of the random forest classifier and are trained by local appearance features. Furthermore, issues such as non-localised spatial support and large inter-subject variability may be dealt with by training with additional data. Even though classification-based methods can be fast, they do not take into consideration organ contextual information or organ shape and as such they often produce less accurate segmentations than registration-based methods.

This paper proposes a novel framework for multi-organ segmentation (Fig. 1(a)), which leverages several ideas from computer vision and machine learning and does not require any registration steps, neither during training nor during segmentation time. Because of this, we can avoid all the potential shortcomings of registration-based methods, while at the same time design a method that is accurate and fast enough that can be applied to real-life clinical applications. We begin by generating supervoxels from the CT image at multiple levels of detail (Sect. 2.1). Then we extract a set of complementary appearance and contextual features from the supervoxels (Sect. 2.2) and use them to train a boosted tree classifier at each level. The classifiers are not independent but are linked together using hierarchical auto-context (Sect. 2.3). During segmentation, the linked classifiers are applied to the new image and their output is fused using a hierarchical conditional random field (Sect. 2.4). We have tested our approach for the segmentation of 8 organs in a 20 CT image dataset (Sect. 3) and obtained results comparable to the state-of-the-art registration-based methods, despite our solution being registration-free. Also, we are considerably more efficient than most competitors since training is done offline and the training data does not have to be present during segmentation. Our key contributions are:

- A method for **registration-free** multi-organ segmentation in 3D CT images
- Multiple levels of **supervoxels** for appearance and context learning
- Adaptation of **auto-context** to a hierarchical scenario
- Extension of **3D feature descriptors** to volumetric data
- **CRF fusion** using spatial and hierarchical supervoxel neighbourhoods

2 Method

2.1 Multi-Level Supervoxels for Learning Appearance and Context

The first step, after acquiring and pre-processing the training data, is to generate a supervoxel representation within which we may extract the appearance features. A supervoxel representation is simply an oversegmentation of the image into homogeneous regions and it is carried out by grouping adjacent voxels based on their intensity similarities. Given a 3D image with voxels $\mathbf{v}=1{:}V$, we can define a supervoxel as the set of voxels $\mathcal{S}_l = \{\mathbf{v} : s(\mathbf{v}) = l\}$, where $l = 1 : L$ and $s : \{1, ..., V\} \rightarrow \{1, ..., L\}$. We have used the fast implementation by [7]. Working with supervoxels is preferable to using single voxels or arbitrary patches, since: (1) we have better adherence to object boundaries and as such are more likely to preserve these boundaries in the final segmentation; (2) The homogeneous regions inside each supervoxel usually come from a single organ since the shape and size of a supervoxel adapts to the local information. Extracting therefore features from inside each supervoxel means that we can capture the specific local structures of individual organs, from a more natural voxel neighbourhood and without confounding information from different organs; Finally, (3) using supervoxels instead of voxels means that we have a reduced model complexity, which in turn results in a much faster algorithm. Instead of using only a single grid to generate the supervoxels, we have adopted a multi-level approach whereby we apply multiple initialisation grids (in a coarse-to-fine strategy), in order to obtain supervoxels at various sizes, shapes and granularity. Our aim with this multi-level approach is to capture a more diverse set of local structures at multiple scales and from different-sized neighbourhoods, in order to obtain a richer representation of organs that may exhibit a large variation in appearance.

2.2   3D Volumetric Feature Extraction

Unequivocally, the most important part of our framework is the choice of features used to train the classifiers, since they directly influence the accuracy of the segmentation. We have extracted a mixture of texture, shape and neighbourhood context features in order to obtain a comprehensive representation of the organs of interest. We denote a feature vector as: $\mathbf{d} = \{\mathbf{d}^{G}, \mathbf{d}^{V}, \mathbf{d}^{H}, \mathbf{d}^{\mathcal{N}}\}$.

3D GLCM features: The gray level co-occurrence matrix (GLCM) is a commonly used approach [8] for extracting statistical features between pixels/voxels in image data. We have adapted this idea to supervoxels, where each entry in the 3D GLCM represents the probability of different graylevels occurring between neighbouring voxels. The neighbourhoods are defined inside a supervoxel and the displacement between two voxels is given by the vector $\{d, \theta, \varphi\}$, where d is the $\mathcal{L}_1$ distance and $\{\theta, \varphi\}$ are the azimuth and zenith angles that determine direction in 3D polar coordinates. For simplicity, we set $d = 1$ and calculated 13 combinations of corresponding directions. This gives 13 Harralick-type features and for each such feature we have extracted both the angular mean and standard deviation, resulting in a 26-dimensional texture vector for every supervoxel.

Volumetric Shape Context Features: The 3D shape context (3DSC) feature [9] is a histogram that accumulates the number of shape points within a given volume. We have extended the 3DSC, originally proposed for 3D point clouds and meshes, to work with volumetric data. We denote this as the Volumetric Shape Context (VSC) descriptor. The VSC uses a 3D gradient intensity histogram centred around each voxel. However unlike the 3DSC, the histogram is now a cube regularly subdivided along its three dimensions, so that each bin describes the same portion of 3D space and contains the same number of voxels. The volume of the cube is given by the volume of the associated supervoxel inside which the current voxel resides. In addition, we assume a global 3D coordinate frame that remains consistent amongst the acquired data. Given thus the gradient $\nabla f(\mathbf{v})$ of a voxel $\mathbf{v}$ at coordinates (v_x, v_y, v_z), each bin $h(k)$ of the histogram stores the average gradient computed from all the N voxels falling within the associated volume of the cube $C(k)$:

$$h(k) = \frac{1}{N} \sum_{\mathbf{v} \in C(k)} \nabla f((v_x, v_y, v_z)). \tag{1}$$

HOG3D Features: The HOG3D is a local descriptor based on oriented histograms of 3D gradients and is complementary to the VSC. We have used the algorithm by [10] and have adapted it to volumetric data and supervoxels. The computation of the descriptor involves first calculating the 3D gradients around a point of interest. Then, the orientation of these gradients is quantised using regular polyhedra and the mean gradient is computed. In our case, the point of interest is the supervoxel centroid. The gradients are computed and averaged over the spatial support of the supervoxel. HOG3D features differ from VSC in that the former uses multiple histograms and accumulates gradient orientations, while the latter has a single histogram and accumulates gradient intensities.

Neighbourhood Context: One simple way of including additional discriminative power into the algorithm is to relate nearby supervoxels together, thereby incorporating neighbourhood context information. This is because in general, the organs of interest have stable relative positions and so we also expect that relative contextual information between supervoxels to be consistent between training and test images. We may define a neighbourhood $\mathcal{N}$ around a given supervoxel $\mathcal{S}_l$ as those supervoxels that share a boundary with $\mathcal{S}_l$. Then for every supervoxel $\mathcal{S}_n$, $n \in \mathcal{N}$ inside the neighbourhood, we calculate the difference $\mathbf{D}_n = \|\mathbf{d}_l - \mathbf{d}_n\|_1$ at each feature-type. Since the size of the neighbourhood can vary for different supervoxels, we only consider the mean and the maximum of $\mathbf{D}_n$, giving us two neighbourhood context features for each supervoxel. Therefore, for every supervoxel we extract a 177-dim vector $\mathbf{d}$, which is composed by concatenating the 26-dim GLCM features $\mathbf{d}^{\mathrm{G}}$ the 125-dim VSC features $\mathbf{d}^{\mathrm{V}}$ the 20-dim HOG3D features $\mathbf{d}^{\mathrm{H}}$ and the 6-dim neighbourhood context features $\mathbf{d}^{\mathcal{N}}$.

2.3   Hierarchical Auto-Context Classification

After feature extraction the next step is to train the classifiers. Here we use the gradient boosted trees (GBT) [11], which is an ensemble prediction method where boosting is applied to weak decision trees. GBTs can often surpass generic random forests and produce a very good fit to the data even in the case of complex nonlinear problems. In order to incorporate all the information contained in the features from the different supervoxels levels, it makes more sense to link the levels together than to treat each level independently. We therefore train one GBT classifier for each supervoxel level and link them using a technique called *auto-context* [12]. In auto-context a classifier is first trained from local features and then applied back onto the image to produce discriminative probability maps. These maps, which act as a rough object localiser, are appended to the existing local features and are used to train a new classifier.

We have introduced two novelties to the basic auto-context algorithm. First, we have extended it to work in a hierarchical scenario and thereby linking together the classifiers from all the levels. More specifically we train the initial GBT from the features extracted at the coarsest level and apply it back onto the image to produce a probability map. The probability map is then transferred to the image on the next level (from coarse supervoxels to fine supervoxels) and together with the features extracted at this new level are used to train a new GBT classifier (Fig. 1(b)). This procedure is repeated until we reach the final level. The output of the training stage is a set of linked GBT classifiers and the output of the segmentation stage is a set of probability maps. The probability maps will be merged in the final CRF fusion step. The second extension is that we further exploit the information in the probability maps and use them as importance sampling weights. Namely, at each subsequent level we only train with the features at locations where the preceding classifier had a high confidence. This step avoids inundating the classifier with too much data and additionally increases the confidence of the classifier at every level by only training with strong, discriminative features.

2.4 Hierarchical CRF Fusion Using Supervoxel Neighbourhoods

The last component of our framework is a conditional random field (CRF) step where the hierarchical outputs from the auto-context classification are fused in order to determine the best labelling. CRF fusion is by far superior to other merging approaches such as voting or averaging. The CRF structure is specified by the undirected graph $\mathcal{G} = (\mathcal{V}, \mathcal{E}_a \cup \mathcal{E}_p)$, where $\mathcal{E}_a = \{(i,j) \in \mathcal{S} \times \mathcal{S} | \ i$ is **adjacent** to $j\}$ and $\mathcal{E}_p = \{(i,j) \in \mathcal{S} \times \mathcal{S} | \ i$ is **parent** to $j\}$. $\mathcal{E}_a$ contains all pairs of supervoxels that are neighbours on the same level, whereas $\mathcal{E}_p$ is the set of all parent-child supervoxel pairs between two subsequent levels. The energy function is given by:

$$E(\mathbf{y}) = \sum_{i \in S} \phi_i(y_i) + \sum_{(i,j) \in \mathcal{E}_a} \phi_{i,j}^a(y_i, y_j) + \sum_{(i,j) \in \mathcal{E}_p} \phi_{i,j}^p(y_i, y_j), \tag{2}$$

where y are the labels. Hence, the CRF introduces both spatial regularisation *within* each level of supervoxels by ϕ^a as well as interaction potentials *between* levels by ϕ^p. We use the probabilistic output $P(y_i|\mathbf{d}_i)$ of the classifiers for the unary potentials:

$$\phi_i(y_i) = -\log P(y_i|\mathbf{d}_i), \tag{3}$$

where $\mathbf{d}$ are the extracted feature vectors we have used to train the classifiers with. The binary potentials are set as:

$$\phi_{i,j}(y_i, y_j; \lambda) = \lambda \exp(-\gamma||\mathbf{d}_i - \mathbf{d}_j||_1)(1 - \delta(y_i, y_j)), \tag{4}$$

with $\gamma = 1/\dim(\mathbf{d})$ and $\delta(.)$ being the Kronecker delta function. λ is a scalar parameter that is chosen separately for the spatial and the hierarchical potentials. We estimate the best labelling $\mathbf{y}^*$ by minimising (2) with the algorithm of [13].

3   Experiments and Results

Dataset: We have used the VISCERAL Anatomy3 dataset [14], which includes 20 contrast enhanced, abdominal CT images. Each CT image has a resolution of 512×512 pixels with an average of 426 slices and a resolution between 0.604–0.793 mm. The images are manually segmented and the ground truth annotations contain up to 20 anatomical structures, albeit not ubiquitous. We will consider 8 organs here: liver, spleen, 2 kidneys, pancreas, 2 lungs, urinary bladder; because they are the most consistently represented in the dataset. In order to improve the appearance learning and discriminative power of the classifier we utilised a secondary add-on dataset, the VISCERAL Silver Corpus [15]. This dataset contains an additional 59 useful CT images, but without any manual ground truth. Instead the labels have been automatically obtained and as such contain segmentation errors. Despite that, the data can still be used for noisy training since the errors are mostly manifested as organ under-segmentations. This means that if we ignore the background information we may still incorporate the partial organ labels from the Silver Corpus.

Pre-processing: Every image was first downsized by a factor of 2 and cropped to speed up training and segmentation. Following that, we converted the data to an isotropic resolution, windowed the Houndsfield units between [0,150] and mapped to intensities in the range [0,1]. Finally, we performed histogram equalisation and denoised the images using 3D anisotropic diffusion.

Training and Segmentation: We defined 9 classes, one for each of the 8 organs and a background class for all the remaining structures. Features were extracted at 4 different levels of detail with 5 k, 10 k, 20 k and 30 k supervoxels respectively. The classifiers were set to run for 300 iterations using an exponential loss function and a tree depth of 2. We followed a leave-one-out evaluation strategy, in which the classifiers were trained on 19(+59 noisy) examples and tested on 1. The final organ labels were obtained by the CRF fusion with fixed parameters $\lambda = 0.05$ for both the hierarchical and spatial potentials.

Results: The main results from our experiments are presented in Table 1 with exemplar segmentation in Fig. 2. We see that our approach obtains good segmentation for the majority of the organs. Furthermore, our results are on par with

Table 1. Jaccard indices of different multi-organ segmentation methods. The numbers have been obtained from their respective publications.

Method	Wang [4]	Chu [2]	Wolz [16]	Oda [3]	Okada [1]	Lombaert [5]	Our	[17]
CT type	?	CTce	CTce	?	CTce	mixed	CTce	CTce
Data size	100	100	150	100	28	250	20	5
Liver	89.57	90.6	88.9	89.0	89.1	73.2	83.68	83.77
R. kidney	85.87	82.3	86.8	80.8	88.2	28.1	86.74	77.30
L. kidney					87.4	29.4	85.37	80.10
Pancreas	48.69	54.6	55.5	42.1	46.6	-	42.30	23.90
Spleen	86.04	84.5	86.2	74.5	82.5	44.5	84.84	65.99
R. lung	-	-	-	-	-	88.4	81.17	92.51
L. lung						85.3	78.20	92.31
Bladder	-	-	-	-	-	-	59.77	60.77

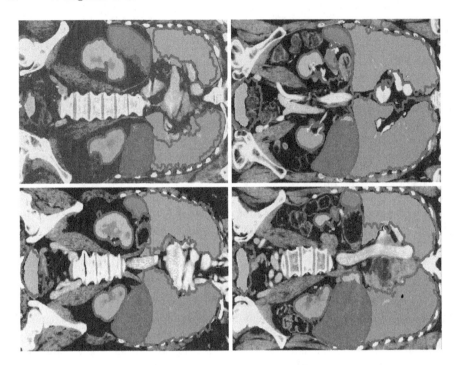

Fig. 2. From left to right: (upper row) Worst, bottom 10 %; (lower row) top 10 % and best results from the 20 evaluated CT images. Our segmentations are outlined in red over the manual labels. (Color figure online)

other state-of-the-art methods from literature that use much larger datasets. Although we cannot yet fully outperform the very accurate registration-based methods [1–4,16] we expect that our results will improve upon increasing the noise-free training data to comparable sizes. Note however that we are considerably better than the classification-based method [5] that does not leverage additional information from the data like we do. For reference, we have also included (last column, Table 1) the average results from the methods participated in the VISCERAL Anatomy2 segmentation challenge [17]. This dataset is closely related to ours and so direct comparison is more reasonable. We observe that our method compares very favourably to the average results reported in [17].

4   Conclusions

We have presented a novel classifier-based framework for registration-free multi-organ segmentation in CT images. We have adapted and extended a number of concepts such as multi-level supervoxels, hierarchical auto-context and CRF fusion, in order to fully leverage all the available information and improve the segmentation quality. Our method was evaluated on a 20 image contrast enhanced CT dataset for the segmentation of 8 organs. In terms of accuracy our results are comparable with other state-of-the-art methods that use a much larger corpus of training data. Also, because our training is done offline and is decoupled from the segmentation stage, we can increase accuracy by training with more data but without any additional segmentation cost. This is not possible for registration-based methods because they do not scale very well with increasing data. Moreover other approaches require all the atlases to be available during segmentation time. All we need to carry over is a small set of trained classifiers with a minimal memory footprint and without data storage and privacy issues. This makes our method efficient, portable and very practical.

References

1. Okada, T., Linguraru, M.G., Yoshida, Y., Hori, M., Summers, R.M., Chen, Y.-W., Tomiyama, N., Sato, Y.: Abdominal multi-organ segmentation of CT images based on hierarchical spatial modeling of organ interrelations. In: Yoshida, H., Sakas, G., Linguraru, M.G. (eds.) Abdominal Imaging. LNCS, vol. 7029, pp. 173–180. Springer, Heidelberg (2012)
2. Chu, C., Oda, M., Kitasaka, T., Misawa, K., Fujiwara, M., Hayashi, Y., Nimura, Y., Rueckert, D., Mori, K.: Multi-organ segmentation based on spatially-divided probabilistic Atlas from 3D abdominal CT images. In: Mori, K., Sakuma, I., Sato, Y., Barillot, C., Navab, N. (eds.) MICCAI 2013, Part II. LNCS, vol. 8150, pp. 165–172. Springer, Heidelberg (2013)
3. Oda, M., Nakaoka, T., Kitasaka, T., Furukawa, K., Misawa, K., Fujiwara, M., Mori, K.: Organ segmentation from 3D abdominal CT images based on atlas selection and graph cut. In: Yoshida, H., Sakas, G., Linguraru, M.G. (eds.) Abdominal Imaging. LNCS, vol. 7029, pp. 181–188. Springer, Heidelberg (2012)
4. Wang, Z., Bhatia, K., Glocker, B., Marvao, A., Dawes, T., Misawa, K., Mori, K., Rueckert, D.: Geodesic patch-based segmentation. In: Medical Image Computing and Computer-Assisted Intervention (2014)
5. Lombaert, H., Zikic, D., Criminisi, A., Ayache, N.: Laplacian Forests: semantic image segmentation by guided bagging. In: Golland, P., Hata, N., Barillot, C., Hornegger, J., Howe, R. (eds.) MICCAI 2014, Part II. LNCS, vol. 8674, pp. 496–504. Springer, Heidelberg (2014)
6. Cuingnet, R., Prevost, R., et al.: Automatic detection and segmentation of Kidneys in 3D CT images using random forests. In: Medical Image Computing and Computer-Assisted Intervention (2012)
7. Holzer, M., Donner, R.: Over-segmentation of 3D medical image volumes based on monogenic cues. In: Proceedings of the CVWW, pp. 35–42 (2014)
8. Kovalev, V.A., Kruggel, F., Gertz, H.J., von Cramon, D.Y.: Three-dimensional texture analysis of MRI brain datasets. IEEE Trans. Med. Imaging $20(5)$, 424–433 (2001)
9. Frome, A., Huber, D., Kolluri, R., Bulow, T., Malik, J.: Recognizing objects in range data using regional point descriptors. In: European Conference on Computer Vision, vol. 3 (2004)
10. Kläser, A., Marszaek, M., Schmid, C.: A spatio temporal descriptor based on 3D Gradients. In: British Machine Vision Conference (2008)
11. Sznitman, R., Becker, C., Fleuret, F., Fua, P.: Fast object detection with entropy-driven evaluation. In: IEEE Conference on Computer Vision and Pattern Recognition (2013)

12. Tu, Z.: Auto-context and its application to high-level vision tasks. In: IEEE Conference on Computer Vision and Pattern Recognition (2008)
13. Komodakis, N., et al.: Performance vs computational efficiency for optimizing single and dynamic MRFs: setting the state of the art with primal-dual strategies. Comput. Vis. Image Underst. **112**(1), 14–29 (2008)
14. Goksel, O., del Toro, O.A.J., Foncubierta-Rodriguez, A., Müller, H.: Proceedings of the VISCERAL Anatomy3 benchmark workshop. In: IEEE International Symposium on Biomedical Imaging, CEUR Workshop Proceedings (2015)
15. Krenn, M., Hanbury, A., Langs, G.: Prototype of silver corpus merging framework (2014)
16. Wolz, R., Chu, C., Misawa, K., Fujiwara, M.: Automated abdominal multi-organ segmentation with subject-specific atlas generation. IEEE Trans. Med. Imaging **32**(9), 1723–1730 (2013)
17. del Toro, O.A.J., Goksel, O., Menze, B., Müller, H., Langs, G., Weber, M., Eggel, I.: VISCERAL VISual Concept Extraction challenge in RAdioLogy: ISBI 2014 challenge organization. In: Goksel, O. (ed.) Proceedings of the VISCERAL Challenge at IEEE International Symposium on Biomedical Imaging, CEUR Workshop (2014)

Structure Specific Atlas Generation and Its Application to Pancreas Segmentation from Contrasted Abdominal CT Volumes

Ken'ichi Karasawa[1(✉)], Takayuki Kitasaka[2], Masahiro Oda[1],
Yukitaka Nimura[1], Yuichiro Hayashi[1], Michitaka Fujiwara[4],
Kazunari Misawa[5], Daniel Rueckert[6], and Kensaku Mori[1,3]

[1] Department of Media Science, Graduate School of Information Science,
Nagoya University, Nagoya, Japan
kkarasawa@mori.m.is.nagoya-u.ac.jp
[2] Department of Information Science, School of Information Science,
Aichi Institute of Technology, Toyota, Japan
[3] Information and Communications, Nagoya University, Nagoya, Japan
[4] Nagoya University Graduate School of Medicine, Nagoya, Japan
[5] Aichi Cancer Center, Nagoya, Japan
[6] Department of Computing, Imperial College London, London, UK

Abstract. Patient-specific atlas is a key technology for the recognition of the human anatomy from 3D medical images. Automated recognition of the pancreas is one main issue for computer-assisted diagnosis and therapy systems in the abdomen because many diseases of the pancreas are not accompanied by noticeable symptoms. In patient-specific atlas generation, hierarchical and mosaicing methods have been proposed to cope with individual differences in the position, orientation, and shape of the pancreas. Even though segmentation accuracy was improved by these methods, it remains lower than for other abdominal organs, such as the liver and the kidneys. The location of the pancreas strongly correlates with the location of vasculature systems, especially the splenic vein. In this paper, we propose a new structure specific atlas generation method that considers the structural information in atlas generation. As for the structural information, we enhance the vasculature using a vesselness filter. Similar volumes in a training dataset with respect to the vasculature structure are selected and used for atlas generation. Using 150 cases of contrast-enhanced 3D abdominal CT volumes, our experiment improved the mis-segmentation of the surrounding organs or such soft tissues as the duodenum.

1 Introduction

Organ segmentation in the abdominal area from 3D medical images is an essential task in abdominal medical image processing. Automated recognition of the pancreas region is one of the main challenges for computer-aided diagnosis and computer-assisted surgery in the abdominal region. The low intensity contrast

© Springer International Publishing Switzerland 2016
B. Menze et al. (Eds.): MCV Workshop 2015, LNCS 9601, pp. 47–56, 2016.
DOI: 10.1007/978-3-319-42016-5_5

among the pancreas and the surrounding organs or soft tissues greatly complicates pancreas segmentation. The intensity information does not effectively support segmentation tasks. Other information is needed, such as the statistical properties on shape and location. Many research groups have tried to segment the pancreas region using probabilistic atlases [1–10]. However, no satisfactory solution has been reported yet because the shape and location of the pancreas have large individual differences. A patient-specific atlas is a more promising approach for pancreas segmentation than a population-specific atlas, which is generated from all the volumes in a dataset. There are unrepresentative shapes in a dataset whose anatomical structures are quite different from the input structure. Thus, we must select shapes that resemble the input image.

Concerning patient-specific atlas generation, hierarchical or mosaicing methods have been proposed [2,3,6,7,9,10]. Hierarchical atlas generation methods have also been proposed [2,3,7,9]. These methods select training atlases from their databases that have similar intensity to that of an input image to generate a patient-specific atlas. However, they only use the image intensity to select similar images. Because the intensity of the soft tissues near the pancreas resembles that of the pancreas region, which is frequently observed in the abdomen region with less visceral fat, atlas selection based on only intensity tends to fail to select similar images from the database. One approach, which utilizes the hierarchical atlas generation method [9], adopts two atlas selection steps. However, both steps are intensity specific atlas selections. Intensity-based atlas selection is also implemented in other research that uses mosaicing techniques [6,10]. Another solution for good pancreas segmentation [5] detects the support structure around the pancreas to build spatial anatomy descriptors. Here, the support structure especially means the position of the vessels around the pancreas. In another work, three types of vessels, the portal vein, the splenic vein, and the superior mesenteric vein, are utilized as support structures to guide pancreas segmentation [5]. Another research proposal localized these vessels to improve the accuracy of pancreas segmentation [11].

In these segmentation methods, they segmented the pancreas regions with better accuracy than the previous methods. However, the accuracy of these methods has not yet reached the level of other abdominal organs' accuracy, for instance, the liver and the kidneys. The location of the pancreas shows strong correlation with that of the vessel structure around it, especially the splenic vein [5,11].

This paper proposes a new atlas generation method to construct subject- and organ-specific probability maps that are generated using selected atlases in a database whose vessel structures around the pancreas resemble those of the input structure. We describe its application in fully automated pancreas segmentation.

The contributions of this paper can be summarized as follows: (1) introduction of structure specific atlas selection for much specific atlas selection, (2) weighted atlas generation using structure specific atlas selection results and intensity-based atlas selection results, and (3) significant improvement of pancreas segmentation by our proposed specific atlas generation scheme.

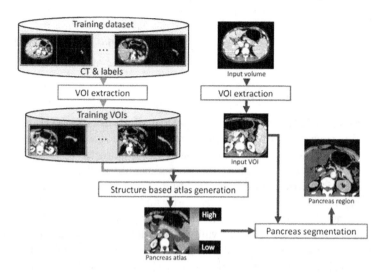

Fig. 1. Flowchart of proposed pancreas segmentation.

2 Structure Specific Atlas Generation and Its Application to Pancreas Segmentation

2.1 Structure Specific Atlas Generation

Such intensity similarities as mutual information and cross-correlation are widely employed in the selection process of similar volumes in a dataset. However, since they evaluate only similarity with respect to the intensity distributions of the volumes of interests, they do not guarantee similarity with respect to anatomical structures. Thus, in patient-specific atlas generation based on the selection of training atlases with similar structures that neighbor the pancreas region, we consider not only the shape and location of a target organ but also the structural information around the pancreas. The location and the structure of the vessels around the pancreas are good anatomical landmarks. We describe the structure specific atlas generation of the pancreas in Sect. 2.3.

2.2 Overview

Our proposed method, which takes the contrasted abdominal CT volume as input and outputs a pancreas region by atlas-based segmentation, consists of three steps: (1) Body size adjustment and pancreas VOI extraction, (2) structure specific pancreas atlas generation, and (3) pancreas segmentation (Fig. 1). The first step includes body size adjustment and pancreas VOI extraction to reduce positional variations of the pancreas among populations. Then we construct a probabilistic atlas for it by selecting training data with similar VOIs to the input VOI with respect to the structure of the vasculature system. After obtaining a patient-specific atlas, we extract the pancreas region by rough segmentation using MAP estimation followed by precise segmentation using the graph-cut technique.

2.3   Pancreas Atlas Generation

(1) Body Size Adjustment and Extraction of Pancreas VOI

Body size adjustment has the following two steps. One is a adjustment of axial plane, and another is a adjustment of head-to-tail direction. To do this, we roughly extract a abdominal region, bottom regions of the kidneys and the lungs using simple region growing and thresholding. Then we adjust the abdominal size of the input image using the average distance between the bottom of the lung regions and the bottom of the kidney regions, and using the average size of abdominal region. These average values are calculated from datasets as pre-process. Then we extract a VOI of the pancreas from the input volume using spatial relationship between ground truth of the liver and of the pancreas to analyze its surrounding structures. The VOI is a rectangular region including the pancreas and its surrounding soft tissues. The VOI location is determined by the centroid of the liver region which is extracted automatically based on a previous method [9]. The VOIs of all the training data are also extracted by the same procedures. We call the VOI of the input volume the *input VOI* and the VOIs of the training data the *training VOIs*. Note that the training VOIs include organ labels that were manually segmented.

(2) Structure Specific Pancreas Atlas Generation

We select 2 N training VOIs that resemble vasculatures around the pancreas of the input VOI in the following two steps. Step 1 (S1) is a selection based on the structure similarity, and Step 2 (S2) is based on the intensity similarity.

In S1, we extract blood vessel (BV) regions by a vesselness filter [12,13] since we focus on the structure of the vasculature system around the pancreas. Noises and unwanted structure such as parts of the spine are eliminated by the morphological opening process. Though thin BVs are also deleted, the thicker ones are sufficient for representing the global structure of the vasculature. Next we calculate the similarity between the BV region of a training VOI and that of the input VOI using zero-mean normalized cross-correlation (ZNCC). We select the top N training VOIs that resemble vessel positions and shapes around the pancreas of the input VOI by the ZNCC measure. The selection is performed before the registration as follows.

We perform MRF-based nonrigid registration [14] between all the training VOIs and the input VOI. In S2, the remaining N training VOIs are selected by the ZNCC value, which is computed based on the intensity value of the VOI. Here, the ZNCC value is calculated after the registration among the images. The BV regions of these selected VOIs are not enhanced by the vesselness filter [12,13].

Finally, we select the 2N training VOIs that were all deformed by the registration. One N training VOI is selected by the ZNCC value, which is calculated in S1. The other N training VOIs are selected by the ZNCC value, which is calculated in S2. To construct a probabilistic atlas, we calculate the weights of the first N training VOIs, w_i^{S1}, and the second N training VOIs, w_i^{S2}, by their ZNCC values. A pancreas atlas is obtained by

$$M_{\mathbf{p} \in V^{(l)}} = \frac{\sum_{i=0}^{N-1} w_i^{S1} w_i^{S2} (\alpha \cdot \delta(L_{1_{\mathbf{p}}}^i, l) + \beta \cdot \delta(L_{2_{\mathbf{p}}}^i, l))}{\sum_{i=0}^{N-1} w_i^{S1} w_i^{S2}}, \tag{1}$$

where $M_{\mathbf{p} \in V^{(l)}}$ is a probabilistic atlas of organ label l for voxel $\mathbf{p}$ in input VOI V. α and β are constants that satisfy $\alpha + \beta = 1$. Here, each organ label l is deformed by the above registration. $\delta(L_{1_{\mathbf{p}}}^i, l)$ and $\delta(L_{2_{\mathbf{p}}}^i, l)$ are delta functions:

$$\delta(l, l') = \begin{cases} 1 \text{ if } l = l', \\ 0 \text{ otherwise,} \end{cases} \tag{2}$$

where $L_{1_{\mathbf{p}}}^i$ and $L_{2_{\mathbf{p}}}^i$ are the organ labels of voxel $\mathbf{p}$ in the i-th VOI of each step.

2.4 Segmentation of Pancreas

Rough segmentation is performed using the probabilistic atlas followed by precise segmentation of the pancreas. We perform its rough segmentation using MAP estimation:

$$l_{\mathbf{p} \in V}^*(\mathbf{x}) = \operatorname*{argmax}_l P_{\mathbf{p} \in V}(\mathbf{x}|l) M_{\mathbf{p} \in V}(l), \tag{3}$$

where $l_{\mathbf{p} \in V}^*(\mathbf{x})$ means an organ label of voxel $\mathbf{p}$ in input VOI V. $\mathbf{x}$ is an intensity value of voxel $\mathbf{p}$ in input VOI V. $P_{\mathbf{p} \in V}(\mathbf{x}|l)$ is the conditional probability of voxel $\mathbf{p}$ given organ label l. EM algorithm [15] estimates term $P_{\mathbf{p} \in V}(\mathbf{x}|l)$ to acquire the rough segmentation result. Finally, precise segmentation is performed using the graph-cut method [16].

3   Experiment and Results

3.1 Dataset

We applied our method to 150 cases of abdominal CT volumes and compared the results with a previous method [9]. These CT scans were acquired from 36 female and 114 male subjects at Nagoya University hospital by a TOSHIBA Aquilion 64 scanner. The subject ages ranged from 26 to 84 with a mean of 62.8 ± 12.0. All the CT scans were obtained for the laparoscopic resection of the stomach, the gallbladder glands, and the colon. The image size, number of slices, pixel spacing, and slice spacing were 512×512 [pixels], 238–1061 [slices], 0.546–0.820 [mm], and 0.4–0.8 [mm], respectively. We evaluated the proposed and previous methods by leave-one-out cross validation by the following four metrics: Jaccard Index (JI), Dice Overlap (Dice), Average Symmetric Surface Distance (ASD), and Root Mean Square Symmetric Distance (RMSD).

Manual segmentations are available for the liver, the spleen, the pancreas, and the kidneys. These gold standards were semi-automatically segmented by three trained raters using region growing or graph-cut segmentation. Let L_1 be a manual segmentation result and let L_2 be an automated result, and these metrics are defined as follows: JI $= |L_1 \cap L_2|/|L_1 \cup L_2|$, DICE $= 2|L_1 \cap L_2|/(|L_1| + |L_2|)$. Higher values of JI and DICE mean greater accuracies. Lower ASD and RMSD values indicate higher accuracies.

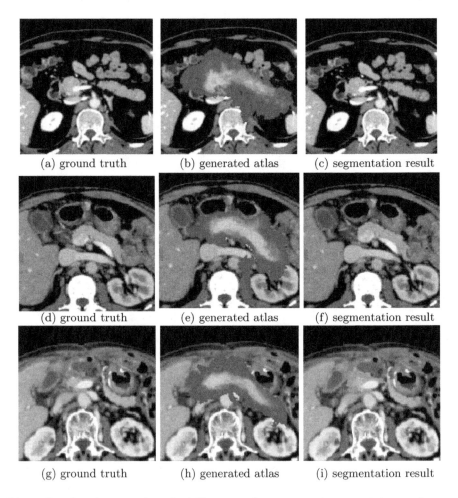

(a) ground truth	(b) generated atlas	(c) segmentation result
(d) ground truth	(e) generated atlas	(f) segmentation result
(g) ground truth	(h) generated atlas	(i) segmentation result

Fig. 2. Results of proposed method. First row shows average segmentation result, second row shows the best one, and third row shows the worst one. JI values were 60.8 %, 78.3 %, and 27.0 %, respectively.

In the experiments, the parameters are $N = 20$, $\alpha = 0.5$, and $\beta = 0.5$. We used Sato's filter [13] as a vesselness filter. This time we only tried $N = 20$ because our proposed method was very time-consuming. We empirically determined that number $N = 20$. Our runtime is described in Sect. 3.2.

3.2 Experimental Results

Our proposed method took about two hours per case, including atlas generation and rough-to-precise segmentation. It took two days on servers equipped with Intel Xeon Dual or a Quad Core $1.86 \sim 3.07$ GHz CPU.

Figure 2 indicates the segmentation results of our proposed method for the average, best, and worst cases. Table 1 shows the accuracy comparison among the proposed method and the state-of-the-art methods of pancreas segmentation [1–10]. Table 1 shows that our proposed method outperformed all other state-of-the-art methods with regard to JI and Dice.

4 Discussion

Figure 3 shows that over-segmentation on the duodenum and the digestive tract was much improved in more than ten cases, although the average accuracy shown in Table 1 just indicates a slight increase. The probabilistic atlases generated by the previous method [9] estimated the duodenum as the pancreas with high likelihood. In contrast, structure specific atlas generation suppressed the estimated duodenum areas as pancreas regions. The JI value of our proposed method improved about twenty points compared to that of the previous one [9] in this case. This is because proper atlas generation was performed based on structure information.

Table 1. Accuracy comparison to other state-of-the-art methods of pancreas segmentation.

Method	# of data	Criteria of pancreas segmentation			
		JI [%]	DICE [%]	ASD [mm]	RMSD [mm]
Shimizu et al. 2010 [1]	98	57.9	-	-	-
Wolz et al. 2013 [2]	150	55.5 ± 17.1	69.6 ± 16.7	3.72 ± 4.36	-
Chu et al. 2013 [3]	100	54.6 ± 15.9	69.1 ± 15.3	1.88 ± 0.64	3.50 ± 1.15
Okada et al. 2013 [4]	86	59.2	71.8	-	-
Hammon et al. 2013 [5]	40	61.2 ± 9.08	-	1.7 ± 0.71	3.10 ± 1.13
Wang et al. 2014 [6]	100	-	65.5 ± 18.6	-	-
Karasawa et al. 2015 [7]	150	60.5 ± 18.1	73.4 ± 17.6	2.10 ± 1.69	3.98 ± 2.63
Roth et al. 2015 [8]	82	-	68 ± 10	-	-
Karasawa et al. 2015 [9]	150	61.3 ± 16.5	74.5 ± 14.9	2.04 ± 1.58	3.86 ± 2.47
Tong et al. 2015 [10]	150	56.9 ± 15.2	71.1 ± 14.7	-	-
Proposed method	150	61.6 ± 16.6	74.7 ± 15.1	1.99 ± 1.47	3.83 ± 2.41

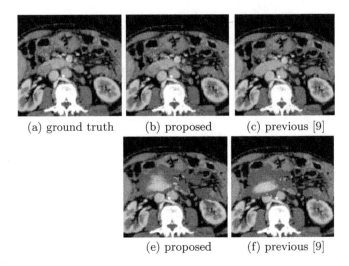

(a) ground truth   (b) proposed   (c) previous [9]

(e) proposed   (f) previous [9]

Fig. 3. Comparison of proposed and previous [9] methods for best case in Fig. 2. First row shows segmentation results and second shows their probabilistic atlases. JI values are 78.3 % and 57.2 %. Previous method segmented the duodenum as well because the probability at the duodenum in the generated atlas has a higher value.

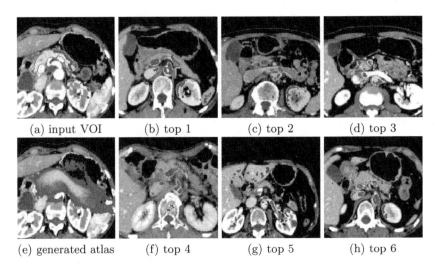

(a) input VOI   (b) top 1   (c) top 2   (d) top 3

(e) generated atlas   (f) top 4   (g) top 5   (h) top 6

Fig. 4. Example of cases in which segmentation accuracy did not increase using our structure specific atlas generation. (a) is the blood vessel enhanced image overlaid on input VOI. (e) is the generated atlas. Top six similar training VOIs are listed in (b-d) and (f-h).

However, in some cases, segmentation accuracy did not improve even with the proposed method. Figure 4 is an example. The images listed in it are the same slice of VOI volumes. Because many unwanted regions enhanced by the vesselness filter were produced in the liver, the kidneys, and the aorta, dissimilar training VOIs were involved in the atlas generation, as shown in Fig. 4 (c,d,g). This produced quite blurry atlases and resulted in the deterioration of segmentation accuracy. The JI values of the proposed and previous [9] methods were 36.8 % and 40.4 %. Improving the extraction of anatomical landmarks for vasculature structure analysis is an important issue to solve.

Compared with other state-of-the-art works [1–8,10], our pancreas segmentation results outperformed the JI and Dice values. Our segmentation accuracy still lags behind [2, 3, 5] for ASD and RMSD values. Note, however, even though the number of datasets used in our experiment is the largest, we obtained the best accuracy values for JI and Dice.

5   Conclusions

We described a structure specific atlas generation method and its application to fully automated pancreas segmentation. The vasculature systems were enhanced by a vesselness filter and used for structural information in atlas generation. As a result of an experiment using 150 cases, over-segmentation of the surrounding organs or such soft tissues as the duodenum was improved, while segmentation accuracy showed just a slight increase from previous methods [9]. Future work will improve the extraction of anatomical landmarks for vasculature structure analysis.

References

1. Shimizu, A., Kimoto, T., Kobatake, H., Nawano, S., Shinozaki, K.: Automated pancreas segmentation from three dimensional contrast enhanced computed tomography. Int. J. Comput. Assist. Radiol. Surg. **5**, 85–98 (2010)
2. Wolz, R., Chu, C., Misawa, K., Fujiwara, M., Mori, K., Rueckert, D.: Automated abdominal multi-organ segmentation with subject-specific atlas generation. IEEE Trans. Med. Imaging **32**(9), 1723–1730 (2013)
3. Chu, C., Oda, M., Kitasaka, T., Misawa, K., Fujiwara, M., Hayashi, Y., Nimura, Y., Rueckert, D., Mori, K.: Multi-organ segmentation based on spatially-divided probabilistic atlas from 3D abdominal CT images. In: Mori, K., Sakuma, I., Sato, Y., Barillot, C., Navab, N. (eds.) MICCAI 2013, Part II. LNCS, vol. 8150, pp. 165–172. Springer, Heidelberg (2013)
4. Okada, T., Linguraru, M.G., Hori, M., Summers, R.M., Tomiyama, N., Sato, Y.: Abdominal multi-organ CT segmentation using organ correlation graph and prediction-based shape and location priors. In: Mori, K., Sakuma, I., Sato, Y., Barillot, C., Navab, N. (eds.) MICCAI 2013, Part III. LNCS, vol. 8151, pp. 275–282. Springer, Heidelberg (2013)
5. Hammon, M., Cavallaro, A., Erdt, M., Dankerl, P., Kirschner, M., Drechsler, K., Wesarg, S., Uder, M., Janka, R.: Model-based pancreas segmentation in portal venous phase contrast-enhanced CT images. J. Digital Imaging **26**(6), 1082–1090 (2013)

6. Wang, Z., Bhatia, K.K., Glocker, B., Marvao, A., Dawes, T., Misawa, K., Mori, K., Rueckert, D.: Geodesic patch-based segmentation. In: Golland, P., Hata, N., Barillot, C., Hornegger, J., Howe, R. (eds.) MICCAI 2014, Part I. LNCS, vol. 8673, pp. 666–673. Springer, Heidelberg (2014)

7. Karasawa, K., Oda, M., Hayashi, Y., Nimura, Y., Kitasaka, T., Misawa, K., Fujiwara, M., Rueckert, D., Mori, K.: Pancreas segmentation from 3D abdominal CT images using patient-specific weighted-subspatial probabilistic atlases. In: Proceeding of Society of Photographic Engineers 9413, Medical Imaging (2015)

8. Roth, H.R., Farag, A., Lu, L., Turkbey, E.B., Summers, R.M.: Deep convolutional networks for pancreas segmentation in CT imaging. In: Proceeding of Society of Photographic Engineers 9413, Medical Imaging (2015)

9. Karasawa, K., Oda, M., Hayashi, Y., Nimura, Y., Kitasaka, T., Misawa, K., Fujiwara, M., Mori, K.: Pancreas segmentation from abdominal CT volumetric images using hierarchically-weighted probabilistic atlases. In: Joint Conference of the International Workshop on Advanced Image Technology and the International Forum on Medical Imaging in Asia, PS.1, 617 (2015)

10. Tong, T., Wolz, R., Wang, Z., Gao, Q., Misawa, K., Fujiwara, M., Mori, K., Hajnal, J.V., Rueckert, D.: Discriminative dictionary learning for abdominal multi-organ segmentation. Med. Image Anal. 23(1), 92–104 (2015)

11. Farag, A., Liu, J., Summers, R.M.: Automatic segmentation of abdominal vessels for improved pancreas localization. In: Proceeding of Society of Photographic Engineers 9037, Medical Imaging (2014)

12. Frangi, A.F., Niessen, W.J., Hoogeveen, R.M., van Walsum, T., Viergever, M.A.: Model-based quantitation of 3-D magnetic resonance Angiographic images. IEEE Trans. Med. Imaging 18(10), 946–956 (1999)

13. Sato, Y., Nakajima, S., Shiraga, N., Atsumi, H., Yoshida, S., Koller, T., Gerig, G., Kikinis, R.: 3D multi-scale line filter for segmentation and visualization of curvilinear structures in medical images. Med. Image Anal. 2(2), 143–168 (1997)

14. Glocker, B., Komodakis, N., Tziritas, G., Navab, N., Paragios, N.: Dense image registration through MRFs and efficient linear programming. Med. Image Anal. 12, 731–741 (2008)

15. Dempster, A.P., Laird, N.M., Rubin, D.B.: Maximum likelihood from incomplete data via the EM algorithm. J. Roy. Stat. Soc. B 39(1), 1–38 (1977)

16. Boykov, Y., Veksler, O., Zabih, R.: Fast approximate energy minimization via graph cuts. IEEE Trans. Pattern Anal. Mach. Intell. 23(11), 1222–1239 (2001)

Machine Learning Based Analyses

Local Structure Prediction with Convolutional Neural Networks for Multimodal Brain Tumor Segmentation

Pavel Dvořák[1,2](✉) and Bjoern Menze[3](✉)

[1] Department of Telecommunications, Brno University of Technology,
Brno, Czech Republic
pavel.dvorak@hotmail.com
[2] ASCR, Institute of Scientific Instruments, Brno, Czech Republic
[3] Institute for Advanced Study and Department of Computer Science,
TU München, Munich, Germany
bjoern.menze@tum.de

Abstract. Most medical images feature a high similarity in the intensities of nearby pixels and a strong correlation of intensity profiles across different image modalities. One way of dealing with – and even exploiting – this correlation is the use of local image patches. In the same way, there is a high correlation between nearby labels in image annotation, a feature that has been used in the "local structure prediction" of local label patches. In the present study we test this local structure prediction approach for 3D segmentation tasks, systematically evaluating different parameters that are relevant for the dense annotation of anatomical structures. We choose convolutional neural network as learning algorithm, as it is known to be suited for dealing with correlation between features. We evaluate our approach on the public BRATS2014 data set with three multimodal segmentation tasks, being able to obtain state-of-the-art results for this brain tumor segmentation data set consisting of 254 multimodal volumes with computing time of only 13 s per volume.

Keywords: Brain tumor · Clustering · CNN · Deep learning · Image segmentation · MRI · Patch · Structure · Structured prediction

1 Introduction

Medical images show a high correlation between the intensities of nearby voxels and the intensity patterns of different image modalities acquired from the same volume. Patch-based prediction approaches make use of this local correlation and rely on dictionaries with finite sets of image patches. They succeed in a wide range of application such as image denoising, reconstruction, and even the synthesis of image modalities for given applications [5]. Moreover, they were used successfully for image segmentation, predicting the most likely label of the

ⓒ Springer International Publishing Switzerland 2016
B. Menze et al. (Eds.): MCV Workshop 2015, LNCS 9601, pp. 59–71, 2016.
DOI: 10.1007/978-3-319-42016-5_6

voxel in the center of a patch [15]. All of these approaches exploit the redundancy of local image information and similarity of *image features* in nearby pixels or voxels. For most applications, however, the same local similarity is present among the *image labels*, e.g., indicating the extension of underlying anatomical structure. This structure has already been used in medical imaging but only at *global level*, where the shape of the whole segmented structure is considered, e.g. [11] or [18]. Here we will focus on *local structure* since global structure is not applicable for objects with various shape and location such as brain tumors.

Different approaches have been brought forward that all make use of the local structure of voxel-wise image labels. Zhu et al. [19] proposed a recursive segmentation approach with recognition templates in multiple layers to predict extended 2D patches instead of pixel-wise labels. Kontschieder et al. [6] extended the previous work with structured image labeling using random forest. They introduced a novel data splitting function, based on random pixel position in a patch, and exploited the joint distributions of structured labels. Chen et al. [2] introduced techniques for image representation using a shape epitome dictionary created by affinity propagation, and applied it together with a conditional random field models for image labeling. Dollar and Zittnick [3] used this idea in edge detection using k-means clustering in label space to generate an edge dictionary, and a random forest classification to predict the most likely local edge shape.

In spite of the success of patch-based labeling in medical image annotation, and the highly repetitive local label structure in many applications, the concept of patch-based local structure prediction, i.e., the prediction of extended label patches, has not received attention in the processing of 3D medical image yet. However, approaches labeling supervoxels rather than voxels has already appeared, e.g. hierarchical segmentation by weighted aggregation extended into 3D by Akselrod-Ballin et al. [1], or spatially adaptive random forests introduced by Geremia et al. [4].

In this paper, we will transfer the idea of *local structure prediction* [3] using patch-based label dictionaries to the task of dense labels of pathological structures in multimodal 3D volumes. Different from Dollar, we will use convolutional neural networks (CNNs) for predicting label patches as CNNs are well suited for dealing with local correlation, also in 3D medical image annotation tasks [7,12]. We will evaluate the local structure prediction of label patches on a public data set with several multimodal segmentation subtasks, i.e., on the 2014 data set of the Brain Tumor Image Segmentation Challenge [9], where a CNN outperformed other approaches [17]. In this paper, we focus on evaluating design choices for local structure prediction and optimize them for reference image segmentation task in medical image computing.

Brain tumor segmentation is a challenging task that has attracted some attention over the past years. It consists of identifying different tumor regions in a set of multimodal tumor images: the whole tumor, the tumor core, and the active tumor [9]. Algorithms developed for brain tumor segmentation task can be classified into two categories: Generative models use a prior knowledge about the spatial distribution of tissues and their appearance, e.g. [13], which requires accurate registration with probabilistic atlas encoding prior knowledge about spatial structure at the organ scale [8]. Our method belongs to the group of *discriminative models*. Such algorithms learn all the characteristics from manually annotated data. In order to be robust, they require substantial amount of training data [20].

In the following, we will describe our local structure prediction approach (Sect. 2), and present its application to multimodal brain tumor segmentation (Sect. 3). Here we will identify, analyze, and optimize the relevant model parameters of the local structure prediction for all different sub-tasks and test the final model on clinical test set, before offering conclusion (Sect. 4).

2   Methods

The brain tumor segmentation problem consists of three sub-problems: identifying the whole tumor region in a set of multimodal images, the tumor core region, and the active tumor region [9]. All three sub-tasks are process separately, which changes the multi-class segmentation task into three binary segmentation sub-tasks.

Local Structure Prediction. Let $\mathbf{x}$ be the *image patch* of size $d \times d$ from image space $\mathcal{I}$. Focusing on 2D patches, a patch $\mathbf{x}$ is represented as $\mathbf{x}(u, v, I)$ where (u, v) denotes the patch top left corner coordinates in multimodal image $I(s, V)$ where s denotes the slice position in multimodal volume V.

Label Patches. Treating the annotation task for each class individually, we obtain a label space $\mathcal{L} = \{0, 1\}$ that is given by an expert's manual segmentation of the pathological structures. The *label patch* is then a patch $\mathbf{p}$ of size $d' \times d'$ from the structured label space $\mathcal{P}$, i.e. $\mathcal{P} = \mathcal{L}^{d' \times d'}$. The label size d' is equal or smaller than the image patch size d. The label patch $\mathbf{p}$ is centered on its corresponding image patch $\mathbf{x}$ (Fig. 1), and it is represented as $\mathbf{p}(u+m, v+m, L)$ where $L(s, W)$ is a manual segmentation in slice s of label volume W and m denotes the margin defined as $m = \frac{1}{2}(d - d')$.

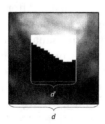

Fig. 1. Local structure prediction: Image feature patches (with side length d) are used to predict the most likely label patch (with side length d') in its center. While standard patch based prediction approaches use $d' = 1$ (voxel), we consider in this paper all values with $1 \leq d' \leq d$.

Optimal values for d and d' and, hence, the ratio $r = \frac{d'}{d}$ may vary depending on the structure to be segmented and the image resolution.

Generating the Label Patch Dictionary. We cluster label patches **p** into N groups using k-means leading to a label patch dictionary of size N. Subsequently, the *label template* **t** of group n is identified as the average label patch of given cluster. In the segmentation process, these smooth label templates **t** are then used for the segmentation map computation rather than strict border prediction as used in previous local structure prediction methods [2,6,19]. The structures are learned directly from the training data instead of using predefined groups as in [19]. Examples of ground truth label patches with their representation by a dictionary of size $N = 2$ (corresponding to common segmentation approach) and $N = 32$ is depicted in Fig. 2.

The size of label patch dictionary N and, hence, the number of classes in the classification problem, may differ between problems depending on variability and shape complexity of the data.

(a)   **(b)**   **(c)**

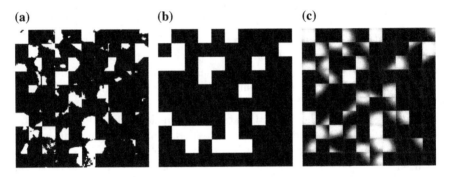

Fig. 2. Ground truth label patches (a) with corresponding binary representation indicating label at the central pixel (b), and structured (c) representation.

Defining the N-Class Prediction Problem. After we have obtained a set of N clusters, we transform our binary segmentation problem into an N class prediction task: We identify each training image patch **x** with the group n that the corresponding label patch **p** has been assigned to during the label patch dictionary generation. In prediction, the label template **t** of the predicted group n (size $d' \times d'$) is assigned to the location of each image patch and all overlapping predictions of a neighborhood are averaged. According to the experiments a discrete threshold $th = 0.5$ was chosen for the final label prediction.

Convolutional Neural Network. We choose CNN as it has the advantage of preserving the spatial structure of the input, e.g., 2D grid for images. CNN consists of convolutional and pooling layers, usually applied in an alternating order. The CNN architecture used in this work is depicted in Fig. 3. It consists of two convolutional and two mean-pooling layers in alternating order. In both convolutional layers, we use 24 convolutional filters of kernel size 5×5. The input of the network is an image patch of size $4 \times d \times d$ (four MR modalities are present in multimodal volumes) and the output is a vector of length N indicating membership to one of the N classes in the label patch dictionary.

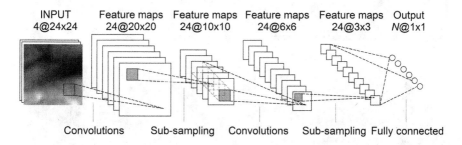

INPUT   Feature maps Feature maps Feature maps Feature maps Output
4@24x24   24@20x20   24@10x10   24@6x6   24@3x3   N@1x1

Convolutions   Sub-sampling   Convolutions   Sub-sampling Fully connected

Fig. 3. Architecture of convolutional neural network for $d = 24$. The input of the network is a multimodal image patch. The output of the network are N probabilities, where N denotes the size of label patch dictionary.

Slice Inference. Image patches from each multimodal volume are mapped into four 2D input channels of the network, similar to RGB image mapping. During the training phase, patches of given size are extracted from training volumes. Using the same approach for testing is inefficient and therefore different approach used in [10] is employed instead. The whole input 2D slice is fed to the network architecture, which leads to much faster convolution process than applying the same convolution several times to small patches. This requires proper slice padding by to be able to label pixels close to slice border.

The output of the network is a map of label scores. However, this label map is smaller than the input slice due to pooling layers inside the CNN architecture. In our case with two 2×2 pooling layers, there is only one value for every 4×4 region. Pinheiro and Collobert [10] fed the network by several versions of input image shifted on X and Y axis and merged the outputs properly. More common approach is to upscale the label map to the size of the input image. The latter approach is faster due to only one convolution per slice compared to 16 using the former approach in our case. Both of them were tested and will be compared.

One can see the sequential processing of the input multimodal slice in Fig. 4. Figure 4(b) and (c) depict 24 outputs of the first and the second convolutional layers of CNN. Figure 4(d) shows the final classification map of the CNN architecture. Note the average labels for given group in Fig. 4(e). One can compare them to the ground truth tumor border in the input image. The final probability map of the whole tumor area is depicted in Fig. 4(f).

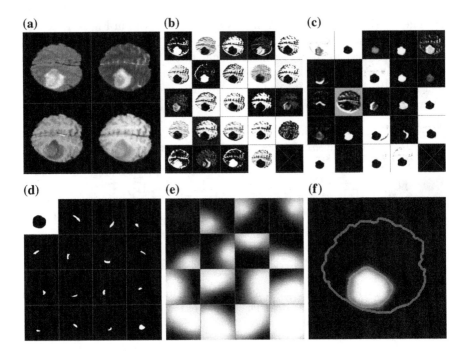

Fig. 4. Sequential processing of multimodal slice (a). (b) and (c) show all 24 outputs of the first and the second convolutional layer. (d) depicts the output of the whole CNN architecture for given 16 groups with average patch labels depicted in (e). (f) shows the final probability map of the whole tumor area with outlined brain mask (blue) and final segmentation (magenta) obtained by thresholding at 50 % probability. (Color figure online)

Since the hierarchy exist between particular segmentation sub-tasks, both tumor core and active tumor are segmented only inside the whole tumor region. This makes the segmentation process much faster. Although the hierarchy exist between tumor core and active tumor as well, this approach is not used here since the segmentation of tumor core is the most difficult sub-task and usually the least accurate one.

Feature Representation. Before the processing of the data, the N4 bias field correction [16] is applied and the image intensities of brain are normalized by their average intensity and standard deviation. All volumes in the BRATS database have the same dimension order and isotropic resolution, therefore the axial slice extraction is straightforward and no pre-processing step to get images in a given orientation and spatial resolution is necessary.

As it has been shown in [12], the computational demands of 3D CNN are still out of scope for today's computers. Therefore, we focus on processing the volume sequentially in 2D in the plane with the highest resolution, in our case the axial plane. Image patches from each multimodal volume are mapped into four 2D input channels of the network. This approach gives a good opportunity for parallelization of this task to reduce the run-time. Alternatives to this basic approach have been proposed: Slice-wise 3D segmentation using CNN was used in [12,14]. The former showed non-feasibility of using 3D CNN for larger cubic patches and proposed using of 2D CNN for each orthogonal plane separately. The later proposed extraction of corresponding patches for given pixel from each orthogonal plane and mapping them as separated feature maps. In our work, we have tested both of these approaches and compared them to the single slice approach that we chose.

3   Experiments

Brain tumor segmentation is a challenging task that has attracted some attention over the past years. We use the BRATS data set that consists of multiple segmentation sub-problems: identifying the whole tumor region in a set of multimodal images, the tumor core region, and the active tumor region [9].

Image Data. Brain tumor image data used in this work were obtained from the MICCAI 2014 Challenge on Multimodal Brain Tumor Image Segmentation (BRATS) training set (http://www.braintumorsegmentation.org). The data contains real volumes of 252 high-grade and 57 low-grade glioma subjects. For each patient, co-registered T1, T2, FLAIR, and post-Gadolinium T1 MR volumes are available. These 309 subjects contain more measurement for some patients and only one measurement per patient was used by us. The data set was divided into three groups: training, validation and testing. Our training set consists of 130 high grade and 33 low grade glioma subjects, the validation set consists of 18 high grade and 7 low grade glioma subjects, and the testing set consists of 51 high grade and 15 low grade glioma subjects, summing up to 254 multimodal volumes of average size $240 \times 240 \times 155$. From each training volume, 1500 random image patches with corresponding label patches were extracted summing up to 244 500 training image patches. The patches are extracted from the whole volume within the brain area with higher probability around the tumor area.

Parameter Optimization. Beside the parameters of the convolutional architecture, there are parameters of our model: image patch size d, label patch size d', and size of label patch dictionary N. These parameters were tested with pre-optimized fixed network architecture depicted in Fig. 3, which consists of two convolutional layers, both with 24 convolutional filters of kernel size 5×5, and two mean-pooling layers in alternating order. The values selected for subsequent experiments are highlighted in graphs with red vertical line.

Image Patch Size. The image patch size d is an important parameter since the segmented structures have different sizes and therefore less or more information is necessary for label structure prediction. Figure 5 shows the Dice score for different patch sizes with their best label patch size. According to the graphs, $d = 8$ was selected for active part segmentation and $d = 24$ for tumor core and whole tumor. All three tests were performed for $N = 32$, which according to the previous tests is sufficiently enough for all patch sizes. The best results were in all cases achieved for $d' \geq \frac{1}{2}d$. The values selected for subsequent experiments are indicated by red vertical line.

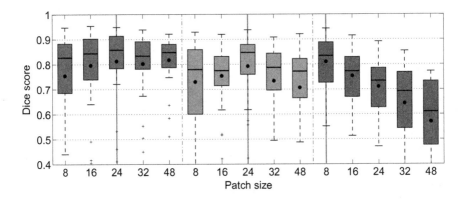

Fig. 5. Dice score as a function of the **image patch size** d with its best label patch size d' with label patch dictionary size $N = 32$ for the whole tumor (blue), tumor core (green) and active tumor (red). (Color figure online)

Size of Label Patch Dictionary. The size of label patch dictionary N influences differences between label each template **t** as well as differences between belonging image patches **x** in each groups n. The results for several values of N are depicted in Fig. 6. Generally the best results were achieved for $N = 16$. The results were evaluated in similar manner as in the previous test, i.e. the best d' is used for each value of N. The values selected for subsequent experiments are indicated by red vertical line. $N = 2$ corresponds to the common pixel-wise approach.

Label patch size. The label patch size d' influences the size of local structure prediction as well as the number of predictions for each voxel. Figure 7 shows the increasing performance with increasing d'. The values selected for subsequent experiments are indicated by red vertical line.

2D versus 3D. We have tested both triplanar and 2.5D deep learning approaches for 3D data segmentation as proposed in [12] and [14], respectively, and compared them to single slice-wise segmentation. For both approaches, we have obtained about the same performance as for single slice-wise approach: the triplanar 2.5D segmentation decreased the performance by 2 %, the 3D segmentation to a decrease of 5 %. This observation is probably caused by lower resolution in sagittal and coronal planes.

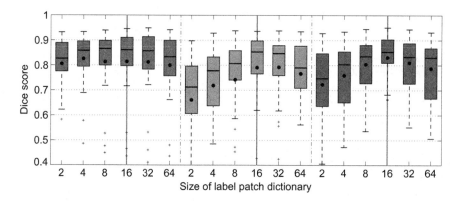

Fig. 6. Dice score as a function of **label patch dictionary size** N using the optima of Fig. 5: $d = 24$ for whole tumor (blue), $d = 24$ for tumor core (green), $d = 8$ for active tumor (red). (Color figure online)

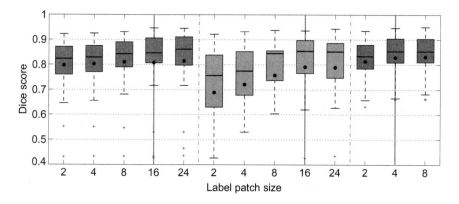

Fig. 7. Dice score as a function of **label patch size** d' for whole tumor (blue) with $d = 24$, tumor core (green) with $d = 24$, and active tumor (red) with $d = 8$, with label patch dictionary size $N = 16$. (Color figure online)

Application to the Test Set. After the optimization of the parameters using validation set, we tested the algorithm on a new set of 66 subjects randomly chosen from BRATS 2014. The performance for both validation and test set of all three segmented structures is summarized in Table 1. For the test set, we achieved average Dice scores 83 % (whole tumor), 75 % (tumor core), and 77 % (active tumor). The resulting Dice scores are comparable to intra-rater similarity that had been reported for the three annotation tasks in the BRATS data set [9] with Dice scores 85 % (whole tumor), 75 % (tumor core) and 74 % (active tumor) and to the best results of automated segmentation algorithms with the Dice score of the top three in between 79 %–82 % (here: 83 %) for the whole tumor segmentation task, 65 %–70 % (here: 75 %) for the segmentation of

Table 1. Segmentation results on validation and test data sets, reporting average and median Dice scores. Shown are the results for all three segmented structures, i.e., whole tumor, tumor core and active tumor. Scores for active tumor are calculated for high grade cases only. "std" and "mad" denote standard deviation and median absolute deviance. HG and LG stand for high and low grade gliomas, respectively.

Dice Score (in %)	Whole	HG/LG	Core	HG/LG	Active
Validation set					
Mean ± std	81±15	80 ±17/85 ± 06	79 ± 13	85 ± 08/65 ± 15	81 ± 11
Median ± mad	86 ± 06	86 ± 07/85 ± 05	85 ± 06	85 ± 03/73 ± 10	83 ± 08
Test set					
Mean ± std	83 ± 13	86 ± 09/76 ± 21	75 ± 20	79 ± 14/61 ± 29	77 ± 18
Median ± mad	88 ± 04	88 ± 03/87 ± 05	83 ± 08	82 ± 07/72 ± 14	83 ± 09

the tumor core, and 58 %–61 % (here: 77 %) for the segmentation of the active tumor region.

We show segmentations generated by our method and the ground truth segmentations for the three regions to be segmented on representative test cases in Fig. 8.

Compute Time vs Accuracy. We have also tested the possibility of subsampling the volume in order to reduce the computational demands. The trade off between accuracy and computing time per volume is analyzed in Table 2 by running several experiments with different resolutions of the CNN output before final prediction of local structure (first column) as well as different distances

Table 2. Tradeoff between spatial subsampling, computing time, and segmentation accuracy. First two columns express different CNN output resolution, i.e., after subsampling in x and y, and steps between segmented slices, i.e., after subsampling in z direction.

CNN output resolution	Slice step	Computing time per volume	Dice score (in%)		
			Whole	Core	Active
1/4	4	13 s	83	75	73
1/4	2	24 s	84	75	74
1/4	1	47 s	84	75	75
1/2	4	22 s	83	75	74
1/2	2	41 s	83	75	76
1/2	1	80 s	84	75	76
1/1	4	74 s	83	75	75
1/1	2	142 s	83	75	77
1/1	1	280 s	83	75	77

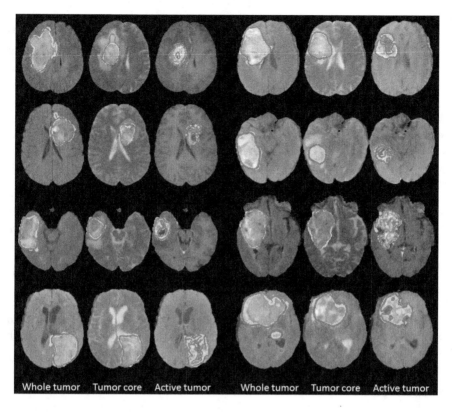

Fig. 8. Example of consensus expert annotation (yellow) and automatic segmentation (magenta) applied to the test image data set. Each row shows two cases. From left to right: segmentation of whole tumor (shown in FLAIR), tumor core (shown in T2) and active tumor (shown in T1c).

between segmented slices (second column), i.e., different sizes of subsequent segmentation interpolation. All experiments were run on 4-core CPU Intel Xeon E3 3.30 GHz. As one can see in the table, the state-of-the-art results can be achieved in an order of magnitude shorter time than in case of most methods participated in BRATS challenge. Thanks to fast implementation of the CNN segmentation, all three structures can be segmented in whole volume in 13 s without using GPU implementation. Processing by the CNN is approximately 80 % of the overall computing time, while assigning final labels using local structure prediction requires only 17 %. The rest of the time are other operations including interpolation. The overall training time, including label patch dictionary generation and training of all three networks using 20 training epochs, was approximately 21 h.

4 Conclusion

We have shown that exploiting local structure through the use of the label patch dictionaries improves segmentation performance over the standard approach predicting voxel wise labels. We showed that local structure prediction can be combined with, and improves upon, standard prediction methods, such as a CNN. When the label patch size optimized for a given segmentation task, it is capable of accumulating local evidence for a given label, and also performs a spatial regularization at the local level. On our reference benchmark set, our approach achieved state-of-the-art performance even without post-processing through Markov random fields which were part of most best performing approaches in the tumor segmentation challenge. Moreover, the all three structures can be extracted from the whole volume within only 13 s using CPU obtaining state-of-the-art results providing means, for example, to do online updates when aiming at an interactive segmentation.

Acknowledgments. PD acknowledges projects SIX CZ.1.05/2.1.00/03.0072, EU ECOP EE.2.3.20.0094, GACR 102/12/1104, and CZ.1.05/2.1.00/01.0017 (ED0017/01/01), Czech Republic. BM acknowledges support through the Technische Universität München-Institute for Advanced Study (funded by the German Excellence Initiative and the European Union Seventh Framework Programme under Grant agreement 291763), and the Marie Curie COFUND program of the European Union.

References

1. Akselrod-Ballin, A., et al.: An integrated segmentation and classification approach applied to multiple sclerosis analysis. In: Computer Vision and Pattern Recognition (CVPR) (2006)
2. Chen, L.C., et al.: Learning a dictionary of shape epitomes with applications to image labeling. In: International Conference on Computer Vision (ICCV), pp. 337–344 (2013)
3. Dollar, P., Zittnick, C.L.: Structured forests for fast edge detection. In: International Conference on Computer Vision (ICCV), pp. 1841–1848 (2013)
4. Geremia, E., Menze, B.H., Ayache, N.: Spatially adaptive random forests. In: IEEE International Symposium on Biomedical Imaging (ISBI), pp. 1332–1335 (2013)
5. Iglesias, J.E., Konukoglu, E., Zikic, D., Glocker, B., Van Leemput, K., Fischl, B.: Is synthesizing MRI contrast useful for inter-modality analysis? In: Mori, K., Sakuma, I., Sato, Y., Barillot, C., Navab, N. (eds.) MICCAI 2013, Part I. LNCS, vol. 8149, pp. 631–638. Springer, Heidelberg (2013)
6. Kontschieder, P., Rota Bulo, S., Bischof, H., Pelillo, M.: Structured class-labels in random forests for semantic image labelling. In: International Conference on Computer Vision (ICCV), pp. 2190–2197 (2011)
7. Liao, S., Gao, Y., Oto, A., Shen, D.: Representation learning: a unified deep learning framework for automatic prostate MR segmentation. In: Mori, K., Sakuma, I., Sato, Y., Barillot, C., Navab, N. (eds.) MICCAI 2013, Part II. LNCS, vol. 8150, pp. 254–261. Springer, Heidelberg (2013)

8. Menze, B.H., van Leemput, K., Lashkari, D., Weber, M.-A., Ayache, N., Golland, P.: A generative model for brain tumor segmentation in multi-modal images. In: Jiang, T., Navab, N., Pluim, J.P.W., Viergever, M.A. (eds.) MICCAI 2010, Part II. LNCS, vol. 6362, pp. 151–159. Springer, Heidelberg (2010)

9. Menze, B., et al.: The multimodal brain tumor image segmentation benchmark (BRATS). IEEE Trans. Med. Imaging (TMI) **34**(10), 1993–2024 (2015)

10. Pinheiro, P.H.O., Collobert, R.: Recurrent convolutional neural networks for scene labeling. In: International Conference on Machine Learning (ICML), pp. 82–90 (2014)

11. Pohl, K.M., et al.: A hierarchical algorithm for MR brain image parcellation. IEEE Trans. Med. Imaging (TMI) **26**(9), 1201–1212 (2007)

12. Prasoon, A., Petersen, K., Igel, C., Lauze, F., Dam, E., Nielsen, M.: Deep feature learning for knee cartilage segmentation using a triplanar convolutional neural network. In: Mori, K., Sakuma, I., Sato, Y., Barillot, C., Navab, N. (eds.) MICCAI 2013, Part II. LNCS, vol. 8150, pp. 246–253. Springer, Heidelberg (2013)

13. Prastawa, M., Bullitt, E., Ho, S., Gerig, G.: A brain tumor segmentation framework based on outlier detection. Med. Image Anal. **8**, 275–283 (2004)

14. Roth, H.R., et al.: A new 2.5D representation for lymph node detection using random sets of deep convolutional neural network observations. In: Golland, P., Hata, N., Barillot, C., Hornegger, J., Howe, R. (eds.) MICCAI 2014, Part I. LNCS, vol. 8673, pp. 520–527. Springer, Heidelberg (2014)

15. Tong, T., et al.: Segmentation of MR images via discriminative dictionary learning and sparse coding: Application to hippocampus labeling. NeuroImage **76**, 11–23 (2013)

16. Tustison, N., et al.: N4ITK: improved N3 bias correction with robust B-spline approximation. In: IEEE International Symposium on Biomedical Imaging (ISBI) (2010)

17. Urban, G., et al.: Multi-modal brain tumor segmentation using deep convolutional neural networks. In: MICCAI-BRATS, pp. 31–35 (2014)

18. Zhang, Y., Brady, M., Smith, S.: Segmentation of brain MR images through a hidden markov random field model and the expectation-maximization algorithm. IEEE Trans. Med. Imaging (TMI) **20**(1), 45–57 (2001)

19. Zhu, L., et al.: Recursive segmentation and recognition templates for 2D parsing. In: Neural Information Processing Systems (NIPS), pp. 1985–1992 (2009)

20. Zikic, D., et al.: Decision forests for tissue-specific segmentation of high-grade gliomas in multi-channel MR. In: Ayache, N., Delingette, H., Golland, P., Mori, K. (eds.) MICCAI 2012, Part III. LNCS, vol. 7512, pp. 369–376. Springer, Heidelberg (2012)

Automated Segmentation of CBCT Image with Prior-Guided Sequential Random Forest

Li Wang[1], Yaozong Gao[1], Feng Shi[1], Gang Li[1], Ken-Chung Chen[2],
Zhen Tang[2], James J. Xia[2,3], and Dinggang Shen[1(✉)]

[1] Department of Radiology and BRIC, University of North Carolina at Chapel
Hill, Chapel Hill, NC, USA
Dinggang_shen@med.unc.edu
[2] Department of Oral and Maxillofacial Surgery, Houston Methodist Research
Institute, Houston, TX, USA
[3] Department of Surgery, Weill Medical College, Cornell University,
New York, NY, USA

Abstract. A major limitation of CBCT scans is the widespread image artifacts such as noise, beam hardening and inhomogeneity, causing great difficulty for accurate segmentation of bony structures from soft tissues, as well as separation of mandible from maxilla. In this paper, we present a novel fully automated method for CBCT image segmentation. Specifically, we first employ majority voting to estimate the initial probability maps of mandible and maxilla. We then extract both the appearance features from CBCTs and the context features from the initial probability maps to train the first-layer of classifier. Based on the first-layer of trained classifier, the probability maps are updated, which will be employed to further train the next layer of classifier. By iteratively training the subsequent classifier and the updated segmentation probability maps, we can derive a sequence of classifiers. Experimental results on 30 CBCTs show that the proposed method achieves the state-of-the-art performance.

1 Introduction

Craniomaxillofacial (CMF) deformities involve congenital and acquired deformities of head and face. The number of patients with acquired deformity is large. In the last decade, the cone-beam computed topographic (CBCT) has become widely used as a valuable technique in diagnosis and treatment planning of patients with CMF deformities due to the lower radiation and lower cost, compared with the spiral multi-slice CT (MSCT). To accurately assess CMF deformities [1], one critical step is to segment the CBCT image to generate a 3D model, which includes segmentation of bony structures from soft tissues, and separation of mandible from maxilla. However, due to the severe image artifacts, including noise, beam hardening, inhomogeneity, and truncation, it is very difficult to segment the CBCT [2]. Moreover, in order to better quantify the deformities, CBCT scans are usually acquired when the maxillary (upper) and mandibular (lower) teeth are in maximal intercuspation, which brings even more challenges to separate the mandible from the maxilla [3].

© Springer International Publishing Switzerland 2016
B. Menze et al. (Eds.): MCV Workshop 2015, LNCS 9601, pp. 72–82, 2016.
DOI: 10.1007/978-3-319-42016-5_7

To date, there is limited work that could effectively segment both maxilla and mandible from CBCT. Manual segmentation is tedious, time-consuming and user-dependent. Previous automated segmentation methods are mainly based on thresholding and morphological operations [4], which are sensitive to the presence of the artifacts [5]. Recently, shape information has been utilized for robust segmentation [6–8], e.g., Zhang et al. [8–10] proposed a deformable segmentation via sparse shape representation. However, these approaches are only applicable to objects with relatively regular shapes (e.g., mandible), but not the objects with complex shapes (e.g., maxilla). Wang et al. [2] proposed a novel patch-based sparse labeling method for automated segmentation of CBCT images with promising results. However, it is computationally expensive (taking hours) due to (1) the requirement of nonlinear registrations between atlases and the target image, and (2) patch-based sparse representation [11–13] for each voxel. Moreover, if a larger number of atlases are used, the computational time becomes even longer. Another limitation is that only simple intensity patches are employed as features to guide the segmentation, which may limit its performance.

Recently, random forest [14] has attracted rapidly growing interest. This approach is a nonparametric method that builds an ensemble model of decision trees from random subsets of features and the bagged samples of the training data, and has achieved the state-of-the-art performance in many image processing problems [15, 16]. In this paper, we present a novel learning-based framework to simultaneously segment both maxilla (along with midface) and mandible from CBCT based on random forest. Our framework is able to integrate information from multi-source images for accurate CBCT segmentation. Specifically, the multi-source images used in our work include the original CBCT images and the iteratively refined probability maps for mandible and maxilla. As a learning-based approach, our framework consists of two stages: (1) training and (2) testing stages. (**1**) In the training stage, we first employ majority voting to estimate the initial segmentation probability maps of mandible and maxilla based on multiple aligned expert-segmented CBCT images. The initial probability maps provide *a prior* guidance for the segmentation [17]. Inspired by the auto-context model [18], we then extract both the appearance features from CBCT and the context features from the estimated probability maps. They are used to refine the segmentations of mandible and maxilla with random forest that can select discriminative features for segmentation. By iteratively training the subsequent classifiers with random forest and auto-context model on both the original CBCT and the updated segmentation probability maps, we can train a sequence of classifiers for CBCT segmentation. (**2**) Similarly, in the testing stage, given a target image, the learned classifiers are sequentially applied to iteratively refine the tissue probability maps by combining previous tissue probability maps with the original CBCT image. We have validated the proposed work on 30 sets of CBCT images. Compared to the state-of-the-art segmentation methods, our method achieves more accurate results.

2 Method

The CBCT scans of 30 patients (12 males/18 females) with nonsyndromic dentofacial deformity, which have been treated with a double-jaw orthognathic surgery, were included in this study. Their ages were 24 ± 10 years (range: 10–49 years).

These CBCT scans were acquired in an i-CAT machine with a matrix of 400 × 400, a resolution of 0.4 mm isotropic voxel, and the time of exposure of 40 s. All the CBCT images were HIPAA de-identified prior to the study. These 30 CBCTs were labeled by one CMF surgeon who is experienced in segmentation using Mimics 10.01 software (Materialise NV, Leuven, Belgium). Even with the help of the tool, it still costs ∼ 12 h per CBCT image. Thus, an automatic method that could effectively and efficiently segment the CBCT images is urgently needed in clinic.

2.1   Prior-Guided Sequential Random Forest

In this paper, we formulate the CBCT segmentation problem as a tissue classification problem. Random forest [14] is adopted here as a multi-class classifier to produce probability maps for each class (i.e., mandible, maxilla, and background) by voxel-wisely classification. The final segmentation is accomplished by assigning the label with the largest probability at each voxel location. As a supervised learning method, our method operates in training and testing stages.

The flowchart of training stage is shown in Fig. 1. In the training stage, **(1)** we first use majority voting to estimate the initial probability maps of mandible and maxilla according to a set of aligned expert-segmented CBCT scans that are used as multi-atlases. **(2)** We then extract both the appearance features from CBCT and the context features from the estimated segmentation probability maps. They are used to refine the segmentations of mandible and maxilla with random forest that can select discriminative features for segmentation. **(3)** To deal with challenges of severe image artifacts and maximal intercuspation (i.e., upper and lower teeth bite closely during CBCT scanning - a clinical requirement for the purpose of accurately quantifying deformities), auto-context model is further adopted to iteratively refine the segmentation probability maps by including context information from the previously-estimated segmentation probability maps to improve CBCT segmentation, especially for separation between mandible and maxilla. **(4)** By iteratively training the subsequent classifiers with random forest and auto-context model on both the original CBCT and the updated segmentation probability maps, we can train a sequence of classifiers for CBCT segmentation. These 4 training steps are summarized in details below.

Step 1: Estimation of Initial Probability Maps with Majority Voting. We employ majority voting to estimate the initial segmentation probability maps of both mandible and maxilla for their rough localizations. In our method, all the expert-segmented CBCT scans will be used as training atlases and further aligned onto the subject CBCT image by affine registration. Then, we employ majority voting to count the votes for each label to estimate the initial probabilities at every voxel. It is simple but robust. The initial probabilities provide spatial priors which are important for guiding the segmentation [15, 17].

Step 2: Extraction of CBCT Appearance and Context Features. We extract these features for training classifiers. Specifically, from CBCT, we extract appearance features, i.e., *random Haar-like features* [19]. From the previous segmentation probability maps, we also extract the context features, which are used to coordinate the

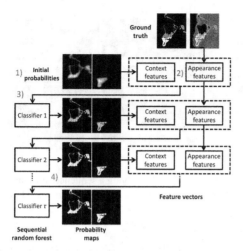

Fig. 1. Flow chart of the proposed training on multi-source: CBCT image, mandible and maxilla probabilities. The appearance features from CBCT images and the context features from iteratively updated probability maps are integrated for training a sequence of classifiers.

segmentations in different parts of CBCT image. This auto-context model has been shown effective in both computer vision and medical image analysis fields [20–23]. For efficiency, we also use *random Haar-like features* [19] to extract context features. Note that, different from the extraction of appearance features, which is performed on un-changed CBCT image, the extraction of context features will be recursively conducted on the updated probability maps.

Step 3: Training of Random-Forest Based Classifiers. To refine the segmentations, we train a classifier to learn the complex relationship between local appearance/context features and the corresponding manual segmentation labels on all voxels of the training atlases. Although many advanced classifiers have been developed in the past, e.g., support vector machine (SVM) [24], random forest [14] is used in our approach because of (1) its effectiveness in handling a large number of training data with high dimensionality, and (2) its fast speed in testing (although slow in training). In addition, random forest also allows us to explore a large number of image features to select the most suitable ones for accurate CBCT segmentation.

Step 4: Repeating Steps 2 and 3 Until Convergence. In this step, we train our classifiers in a serial manner. Specifically, based on the classifier trained in Step 3, we can update the segmentation probability maps. Then, according to Step 2, we can extract the context features from the updated segmentation probability maps, and further use with the original CBCT appearance features to train a next classifier. Eventually, we train and obtain a sequence of classifiers for CBCT segmentation.

In the testing stage, given a new CBCT image, as shown in Fig. 2(a), the corresponding probability maps of mandible and maxilla can be estimated by using the

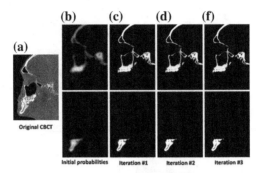

Fig. 2. The estimated probability maps by applying a sequence of trained classifier on an unseen CBCT image (a). The probability maps become more accurate and sharper along the iterations (b–e).

serial trained classifiers. Specifically, as in Step 1 of training stage, the initial segmentation probability maps of mandible and maxilla are first estimated using majority voting (Fig. 2(b)). Then, based on the estimated probability maps, the context features are extracted and, together with CBCT appearance features, served as the input to the serial classifiers for iteratively updating the segmentation probability maps. Based on the output of the serial classifiers, the new CBCT image is finally segmented. As we can see from Fig. 2(b–e), the probability maps are updated with the iterations and becoming more and more accurate.

3   Experimental Results

In our implementation, we smooth the initial probability maps by a Gaussian filter with $\sigma = 2$ mm [25]. For each class, we select 5000 training voxels from each image. Then, from $27 \times 27 \times 27$ patch of each training voxel, 10,000 random Haar features are extracted from all source images/maps: CBCT images, and probability maps of mandible, maxilla and background. For each iteration, we train 40 deep classification trees. We stop the tree growth at a certain depth ($d = 100$), or with the condition that no tree leaf contains less than a certain number of samples ($s_{min} = 8$), according to [25].

The validation is performed on 30 CBCT subjects in a leave-one-out strategy. In the following, we first demonstrate the importance of prior and sequential random forest. Then we make qualitative and quantitative comparisons with the state-of-the-art methods.

Importance of Prior and Sequential Random Forest. Figure 3 shows the Dice ratios on 30 isointense subjects by applying a sequence of classifiers. The green and red curves are the results by the sequential random forest without and with prior, respectively. At the beginning (#0 iteration), the Dice ratios are calculated on the results by majority voting, which provides the prior for the sequential random forest. For the sequential random forest with prior, along the iterations, it can be seen that the Dice ratios are increasing and become stable after a few iterations. By contrast, for the

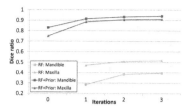

Fig. 3. The Dice ratios of mandible and maxilla on 30 CBCT subjects by the sequential random forest without (green curves) and with prior (red curves). (Color figure online)

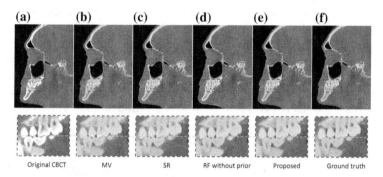

Fig. 4. Comparisons of segmentation results of different methods on (a) a typical CBCT image: (b) majority voting (MV), (c) patch-based sparse representation (SR) [2], (d) sequential random forest without prior [16], (e) the proposed sequential random forest with prior, and (f) ground truth.

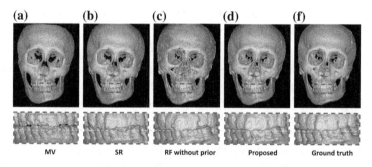

Fig. 5. 3D surfaces obtained by different methods: (a) majority voting (MV), (b) patch-based sparse representation (SR) [2], (c) sequential random forest without prior [16], (d) the proposed sequential random forest with prior, and (e) ground truth.

sequential random forest without prior, its results are much worse than the results with prior. The primary reason is due to the similar bony appearances shared by mandible, maxilla and cervical vertebrae. Without the spatial prior, they could be mislabeled, as observed in Fig. 4(d) and 5(c). This comparison clearly demonstrates the importance of using (1) the prior in guiding the CBCT segmentation and (2) sequential random forest in further improving the accuracy.

Comparisons with the State-of-the-Art Methods. Figure 4 presents the segmentation results on a slice using different methods for one typical subject. From left to right, the first row shows the original CBCT image, and the results obtained by majority voting (MV), patch-based sparse representation (SR) [2], sequential random forest without prior, the proposed sequential random forest with prior, and the manual segmentation. The second row shows the zoomed views for better visualization. Due to possible error during affine registration, the result by MV is not accurate, which, however, is adequate to provide a prior. For the SR, to achieve the best performance, we have applied a nonlinear registration method (Elastix) [26] to align all atlases to the target subject. However, due to the closed-bite position and large intensity variations, the SR [2] still cannot accurately separate the mandible from the maxilla. Without prior, the sequential random forest [16] mislabels the mandible and maxilla, as indicated by the red arrows. While the proposed prior-guided sequential random forest achieves a reasonable result, which is much consistent with the ground truth. The corresponding 3D surfaces generated by different methods are shown in Fig. 5, which also clearly demonstrates more consistency of our result with the ground truth than others. Moreover, the proposed prior-guided sequential random forest only requires ∼ 20 min (i.e., 5 min for MV plus 15 min for prior-guided sequential random forest) for segmentation of a typical CBCT image, as listed in Table 1. By contrast, the SR requires hours. Remember that the manual segmentation usually costs ∼ 12 h for every CBCT image. Therefore, our proposed method will be able to greatly improve the efficiency in clinic.

We then quantitatively evaluate the performance of different methods, as shown in Table 1. Using prior and the sequential random forest, the proposed method achieves the highest Dice ratios. To further validate the proposed method, we also evaluate the accuracy by measuring the average surface distance error, which is defined as: $D(A, B) = \frac{1}{2} \left(\frac{1}{n_A} \sum_{a \in surf(A)} dist(a, B) + \sum_{b \in surf(B)} dist(b, A) \right)$, where $surf(A)$ is the surface of segmentation A, n_A is the total number of surface points in $surf(A)$, and $dist(a, B)$ is the Euclidean distance between a surface point a and the nearest surface point of segmentation B. Additionally, the Hausdorff distance was also used to measure the maximal surface-distance errors of each of 30 subjects. The average surface distance and Hausdorff distance on all 30 subjects are shown in Table 1, which again demonstrates the advantage of our proposed method.

To further demonstrate the advantages of the proposed method in terms of separation of lower and upper teeth, Figs. 6 and 7 show the results by different methods on the teeth part (the incisors and canines & molars) from 7 different subjects. The appearance varies from open-mouth to closed-bite in MI. It indicates that the proposed method can achieve more accurate results than SR [1], especially for the close-bite cases. We also

Table 1. Average dice ratios and surface distance errors (in mm) on 30 subjects.

		MV	SR [2]	RF without prior [16]	Proposed (RF with prior)
Running time		5 m	5 h	15 m	20 m
Dice ratio	Mandible	0.83 ± 0.04	0.92 ± 0.03	0.51 ± 0.12	**0.94 ± 0.02**
	Maxilla	0.75 ± 0.04	0.88 ± 0.02	0.39 ± 0.14	**0.91 ± 0.03**
Average distance	Mandible	1.21 ± 0.25	0.62 ± 0.23	3.42 ± 1.21	**0.42 ± 0.15**
Hausdorff distance	Mandible	3.65 ± 1.53	0.95 ± 0.24	4.74 ± 2.56	**0.74 ± 0.25**

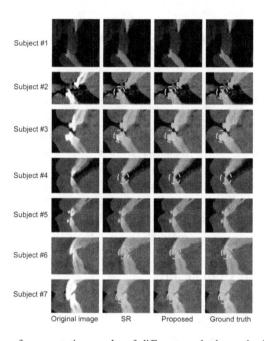

Fig. 6. Comparisons of segmentation results of different methods on the incisors part from 7 typical CBCTs.

quantitatively measured the performance in the teeth part via Dice ratios, average surface distance, and Hausdorff distance. The measurements are shown in Table 2, in which our method achieves significantly better results than SR [1] (p-value < 0.001).

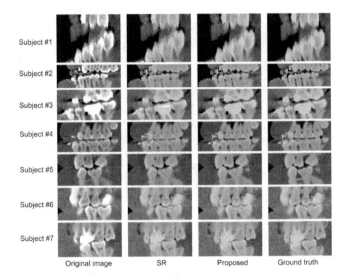

Fig. 7. Comparisons of segmentation results of different methods on the canines and molars part from 7 typical CBCTs.

Table 2. Average dice ratios and surface distance errors (in mm) for the teeth part from 30 CBCTs.

		SR [2]	Proposed
Dice ratio	Mandible	0.915 ± 0.024	0.958 ± 0.016
	Maxilla	0.893 ± 0.028	0.926 ± 0.021
Average distance	Mandible	0.723 ± 0.343	0.312 ± 0.103
	Maxilla	0.739 ± 0.411	0.346 ± 0.154
Hausdorff distance	Mandible	1.266 ± 0.316	0.618 ± 0.186
	Maxilla	1.361 ± 0.352	0.669 ± 0.209

4   Discussion and Conclusion

We have developed and validated a novel fully automated method for CBCT segmentation. We first estimate initial probability maps for mandible and maxilla, to provide a prior for the subsequent classifier training. We then extract both appearance features from CBCT and the context features from the initial probability maps to train the first-layer classifier via random forest. The first-layer classifier returns new probability maps. To deal with challenges of severe image artifacts and maximal inter-cuspation, inspired by the auto-context model, the updated probability maps, together with the original CBCT features, are iteratively used to guide the training of the next classifier in the next round of training. Finally, a sequence of classifiers is learned. We have validated our proposed method on 30 CBCT subjects with promising results.

In our current work, considering the computational time and robustness, we employ just majority voting to estimate the initial prior for our prior-guided sequential random forest. Although it may be more reasonable to use the results by the SR [2] as prior due to their higher accuracy than majority voting, the computation of SR is expensive. Also, even with the low accuracy of majority voting, the proposed sequential random forest still achieves better performance than the SR.

References

1. Wang, L., Ren, Y., Gao, Y., Tang, Z., Chen, K.C., Li, J., Shen, S.G., Yan, J., Lee, P.K., Chow, B., Xia, J.J., Shen, D.: Estimating patient-specific and anatomically correct reference model for craniomaxillofacial deformity via sparse representation. Med. Phys. **42**, 5809 (2015)
2. Wang, L., Chen, K.C., Gao, Y., Shi, F., Liao, S., Li, G., Shen, S.G.F., Yan, J., Lee, P.K.M., Chow, B., Liu, N.X., Xia, J.J., Shen, D.: Automated bone segmentation from dental CBCT images using patch-based sparse representation and convex optimization. Med. Phys. **41**, 043503 (2014)
3. Le, B.H., Deng, Z., Xia, J., Chang, Y.-B., Zhou, X.: An interactive geometric technique for upper and lower teeth segmentation. In: Yang, G.-Z., et al. (eds.) MICCAI 2009, vol. 5762, pp. 968–975. Springer, Berlin Heidelberg (2009)
4. Hassan, B.A.: Applications of Cone Beam Computed Tomography in Orthodontics and Endodontics. Thesis, Reading University, VU University Amsterdam (2010)
5. He, L., Zheng, S.F., Wang, L.: Integrating local distribution information with level set for boundary extraction. J. Vis. Commun. Image Represent. **21**, 343–354 (2010)
6. Kainmueller, D., Lamecker, H., Seim, H., Zinser, M., Zachow, S.: Automatic extraction of mandibular nerve and bone from cone-beam CT data. In: Yang, G.-Z., et al. (eds.) MICCAI 2009, vol. 5762, pp. 76–83. Springer, Heidelberg (2009)
7. Gollmer, S.T., Buzug, T.M.: Fully automatic shape constrained mandible segmentation from cone-beam CT data. In: ISBI, pp. 1272–1275 (2012)
8. Zhang, S., Zhan, Y., Dewan, M., Huang, J., Metaxas, D.N., Zhou, X.S.: Deformable segmentation via sparse shape representation. In: Fichtinger, G., et al. (eds.) MICCAI 2011, vol. 6892, pp. 451–458. Springer, Heidelberg (2011)
9. Zhang, S., Zhan, Y., Dewan, M., Huang, J., Metaxas, D.N., Zhou, X.S.: Towards robust and effective shape modeling: sparse shape composition. Med. Image Anal. **16**, 265–277 (2012)
10. Zhang, S.T., Zhan, Y.Q., Metaxas, D.N.: Deformable segmentation via sparse representation and dictionary learning. Med. Image Anal. **16**, 1385–1396 (2012)
11. Wang, L., Shi, F., Gao, Y., Li, G., Gilmore, J.H., Lin, W., Shen, D.: Integration of sparse multi-modality representation and anatomical constraint for isointense infant brain MR image segmentation. NeuroImage **89**, 152–164 (2014)
12. Wang, L., Shi, F., Li, G., Gao, Y., Lin, W., Gilmore, J.H., Shen, D.: Segmentation of neonatal brain MR images using patch-driven level sets. NeuroImage **84**, 141–158 (2014)
13. Shi, F., Wang, L., Wu, G.R., Li, G., Gilmore, J.H., Lin, W.L., Shen, D.: Neonatal atlas construction using sparse representation. Hum. Brain Mapp. **35**, 4663–4677 (2014)
14. Breiman, L.: Random forests. Mach. Learn. **45**, 5–32 (2001)
15. Zikic, D., Glocker, B., Criminisi, A.: Encoding atlases by randomized classification forests for efficient multi-atlas label propagation. Med. Image Anal. **18**, 1262–1273 (2014)
16. Wang, L., Gao, Y., Shi, F., Li, G., Gilmore, J.H., Lin, W., Shen, D.: LINKS: learning-based multi-source integration framework for segmentation of infant brain images. NeuroImage **108**, 160–172 (2015)

17. Zikic, D., Glocker, B., et al.: Decision forests for tissue-specific segmentation of high-grade gliomas in multi-channel MR. In: Ayache, N., et al. (eds.) Medical Image Computing and Computer-Assisted Intervention – MICCAI 2012, vol. 7512, pp. 369–376. Springer, Heidelberg (2012)
18. Tu, Z., Bai, X.: Auto-context and its application to high-level vision tasks and 3D brain image segmentation. IEEE Trans. Pattern Anal. Mach. Intell. **32**, 1744–1757 (2010)
19. Viola, P., Jones, M.J.: Robust real-time face detection. Int. J. Comput. Vis. **57**, 137–154 (2004)
20. Sutton, C., McCallum, A., Rohanimanesh, K.: Dynamic conditional random fields: factorized probabilistic models for labeling and segmenting sequence data. J. Mach. Learn. Res. **8**, 693–723 (2007)
21. Oliva, A., Torralba, A.: The role of context in object recognition. Trends Cogn. Sci. **11**, 520–527 (2007)
22. Belongie, S., Malik, J., Puzicha, J.: Shape matching and object recognition using shape contexts. IEEE Trans. Pattern Anal. Mach. Intell. **24**, 509–522 (2002)
23. Geman, S., Geman, D.: Stochastic relaxation, Gibbs distributions, and the Bayesian restoration of images. IEEE Trans. Pattern Anal. Mach. Intell. **6**, 721–741 (1984)
24. Hsu, C.-W., Lin, C.-J.: A comparison of methods for multiclass support vector machines. IEEE Trans. Neural Netw. **13**, 415–425 (2002)
25. Zikic, D., Glocker, B., Criminisi, A.: Atlas encoding by randomized forests for efficient label propagation. In: Mori, K., et al. (eds.) Medical Image Computing and Computer-Assisted Intervention – MICCAI 2013, vol. 8151, pp. 66–73. Springer, Berlin Heidelberg (2013)
26. Klein, S., Staring, M., Murphy, K., Viergever, M.A., Pluim, J.: Elastix: a toolbox for intensity-based medical image registration. IEEE Trans. Med. Imaging **29**, 196–205 (2010)

Subject-Specific Estimation of Missing Cortical Thickness Maps in Developing Infant Brains

Yu Meng[1,2], Gang Li[2], Yaozong Gao[1,2], John H. Gilmore[2],
Weili Lin[2], and Dinggang Shen[2(✉)]

[1] Department of Computer Science, University of North Carolina at Chapel Hill,
Chapel Hill, NC, USA
[2] Department of Radiology and BRIC,
University of North Carolina at Chapel Hill, Chapel Hill, NC, USA
dgshen@med.unc.edu

Abstract. To accurately chart the dynamic brain developmental trajectories in infants, many longitudinal neuroimaging studies prefer having a complete dataset. Unfortunately, missing data at certain time points are unavoidable in longitudinal datasets. To better use incomplete longitudinal data, we propose a novel method to estimate the subject-specific vertex-wise cortical thickness maps at missing time points, by using a customized regression forest, Dynamically-Assembled Regression Forest (DARF). DARF ensures spatial smoothness of the estimated cortical thickness maps and also the computational efficiency. The proposed method can fully exploit the available information from the subjects both with and without missing scans. Our method has been applied to estimate the missing cortical thickness maps in a longitudinal infant dataset, which includes 31 healthy subjects, with each having up to 5 scans. The experimental results indicate that our method can accurately estimate missing cortical thickness maps, with the average vertex-wise error less than 0.23 mm.

Keywords: Missing data completion · Longitudinal cortical thickness · Infant brain development

1 Introduction

In recent years, longitudinal neuroimaging analysis of early postnatal brain development has received increasing attention [1–5], because this can capture both the subject-specific and population-averaged dynamic developmental trajectories of the cerebral cortex. This will help better understand the relationship between normal structural and functional development of the cerebral cortex [6–9], and will also provide important references for understanding of many neurodevelopmental disorders, which are likely caused by the abnormal early brain development [1, 10]. To accurately chart the dynamic early brain developmental trajectories, many studies prefer using the subjects with complete longitudinal scans. However, in longitudinal studies, as shown in Fig. 2(a), missing data at certain time points are unavoidable due to various reasons, such as subject absence from scheduled scans or poor imaging quality. Directly using incomplete longitudinal data would introduce biases and also reduce precision and

© Springer International Publishing Switzerland 2016
B. Menze et al. (Eds.): MCV Workshop 2015, LNCS 9601, pp. 83–92, 2016.
DOI: 10.1007/978-3-319-42016-5_8

power in statistical analysis, while discarding subjects with missing data would cause a terrible waste of potentially useful information and also the considerable cost for data acquisition. Owing to the highly dynamic and nonlinear development of the infant brain, a simple linear interpolation or regression cannot accurately estimate the missing data. Although several other methods have been proposed to estimate or complete the missing data for general purpose [11, 12], their effectiveness reduces with the increase of the portion of missing data. To deal with large portion of missing data, the low rank matrix completion methods have been proposed [13, 14]; however, they work well only if the missing data are distributed randomly and uniformly. Thus, the existing methods are not suitable for estimation of regionally-heterogeneous and longitudinally-dynamic cortical thickness map in infant brain studies.

To bridge this critical gap, in this paper, we unprecedentedly propose a novel general learning-based framework for subject-specific estimation of the vertex-wise *cortical thickness* map at the missing time point(s) in longitudinal infant brain studies. Of note, cortical thickness is an important macroscopic morphological measure of the cerebral cortex in MRI studies, and changes of CT are found in normal development, aging, and brain disorders, indicating differential underlying microstructural changes of the cortex in different states [10]. Technically, we propose a Dynamically-Assembled Regression Forest (DARF), a customized version of random forest, as our core regression tool. By sharing decision trees with neighboring forests, DARF ensures spatial smoothness of the vertex-wise regression/estimation result and also greatly reduces the training time, compared to the conventional regression forest. Hereafter, we refer the vertex-wise cortical thickness maps at missing time points as missing data. To fully exploit the information of both the subjects with complete longitudinal data and the subjects with missing data, our method contains two major stages. In the first stage, to use as many training subjects as possible, the missing data at each time point of each subject is estimated *multiple times* based on the data at different available time points *independently*, and then these estimated results are averaged as the initial estimation. In the second stage, to better capitalize on longitudinal information and make the estimations temporally consistent, the missing data at each time point of each subject is refined based on both the real data and the initially estimated missing data at all the other time points *jointly*. As shown in the experiments, our method can accurately estimate the subject-specific cortical thickness map at missing time points in longitudinal infant studies, with the average vertex-wise error less than 0.23 mm.

2   Methods

In this section, we first introduce our regression model, namely Dynamically-Assembled Random Forest (DARF), and then describe how to use this regression model for subject-specific estimation of vertex-wise cortical thickness map at the missing time point(s) in longitudinal infant studies. Of note, before the estimation of missing data, the longitudinal cortical surfaces of all infants were reconstructed [15] and warped onto the same *spherical* space to establish both intra-subject and inter-subject cortical correspondences, and subsequently all cortical surfaces were resampled to have the same triangular mesh configuration using a method similar to [16]. Cortical thickness and sulcal depth were computed for each vertex on each cortical surface [15, 16].

2.1 Dynamically-Assembled Regression Forest

Motivation. We adopt regression forest [17] as our core regression tool. However, using only one conventional regression forest (CRF) cannot accurately estimate vertex-wise cortical thickness maps, because cortical thickness and its developmental patterns are both regionally heterogeneous. An intuitive way to solve this issue is to first divide the cortical surface into a set of small regions of interest (ROIs), and then train a specific regression forest for each ROI. However, this will lead to spatially unsmooth estimation results around the boundaries of neighboring ROIs, since the cortical thicknesses of the vertices near to the ROI boundary are estimated using two completely different regression forests, which are trained independently with different training samples. Although using the highly overlapped ROIs could produce relatively smooth estimation results, it requires a large set of ROIs to uniformly cover the whole cortex, and thus leads to large computational workload. To address these issues, we proposed a Dynamically-Assembled Regression Forest (DARF). By sharing large portions of trees with the neighboring forests, DARF can make the estimation result as smooth as the real data, and also greatly reduce the training time.

Training and Testing. In the training stage, an individual binary decision tree is trained at each vertex on the spherical surface. Specifically, as shown in Fig. 1(a), for a given vertex, all its nearby vertices in a specified neighborhood (i.e., red region) on the spherical cortical surface are used as training samples. For each training sample i, we have a feature vector $X_i \in \mathbb{R}^d$, and a regression response $y_i \in \mathbb{R}$. The feature vector X_i consists of a set of features (see Sect. 2.2) extracted from the local cortical attribute (e.g., cortical thickness and sulcal depth) maps at input time points, and the regression response y_i is the cortical thickness value at the target time point. In the testing stage, to estimate the cortical thickness at a given vertex, as shown in Fig. 1(b), all the nearby individual trees trained for vertices in a specified neighborhood (i.e., green region) are grouped together to form a DARF. Then the feature vector of the given vertex is fed to the DARF to estimate the cortical thickness at the target time point.

Smoothness. DARF is able to produce spatially very smooth estimations, because (1) the DARFs of neighboring vertices are very similar, as they share a large number of trees, and (2) the features of neighboring vertices are also similar.

2.2 Feature Computation on Spherical Surface

For each vertex i, its feature vector $X_i \in \mathbb{R}^d$ includes two types of features: local features and context features. Herein, local features provide localized information at each vertex, while context features provide rich neighboring information. In our implementation, local features are the cortical thickness and sulcal depth. The context

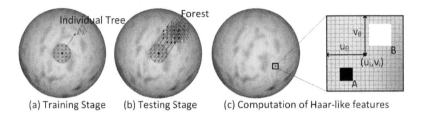

(a) Training Stage   (b) Testing Stage   (c) Computation of Haar-like features

Fig. 1. Illustration of training and testing stages of DARF, and also the computation of Haar-like features on a spherical surface. In (a), the red region is the neighborhood, where all the vertices are used as training samples. In (b), the green region is the neighborhood, where all trained individual trees are assembled as a forest. Note that the red and green regions can be in different sizes. In (c), the white and black blocks are the two randomly selected regions for computing Haar-like features. (Color figure online)

features are a set of randomly defined Haar-like features, which provide two types of context information: (1) the mean attributes (i.e., cortical thickness and sulcal depth) in a small cortical region, and (2) the difference between mean attributes in two small regions. The computation of Haar-like features on spherical surfaces is shown in Fig. 1 (c). Specifically, given a vertex (u_i, v_i), where u_i and v_i are respectively the latitude and longitude coordinates, two blocks A and B are randomly selected in the neighborhood $[u_i \pm u_\theta, v_i \pm v_\theta]$, and their sizes are also randomly chosen from the interval $[r_1, r_2]$, where u_θ, v_θ, r_1, and r_2 are the user-defined parameters. Let S_a and S_b denote the sets of all the vertices in blocks A and B, respectively, and then the Haar-like features at the vertex (u_i, v_i) can be mathematically formulated as:

$$f(u_i, v_i) = \frac{1}{|S_a|} \sum_{(u,v) \in S_a} M(u, v) - \lambda \frac{1}{|S_b|} \sum_{(u,v) \in S_b} M(u, v) \qquad (1)$$

where $M(u, v)$ is the value of cortical morphological attributes (i.e., cortical thickness and sulcal depth) at vertex (u, v), and λ is a random coefficient that can only be 0 or 1. In the case of $\lambda = 0$, Haar-like feature is the mean value of the cortical attribute within the block A. In the case of $\lambda = 1$, Haar-like feature is the difference betweenthe mean values of the cortical attribute in the block A and block B.

2.3   Estimation of Cortical Thickness Maps at Missing Time Points

Figure 2(a) shows the longitudinal infant dataset with missing data used in this paper, which includes 31 subjects (with 15 subjects having missing data), each subject with up to 5 time points in the first postnatal year. Intuitively, using the data at multiple available time points to estimate the missing ones is better than using the data at just one available time point, because multiple time points capture more information of the nonlinear longitudinal cortex development in infants. However, owing to the missing data, as shown in Fig. 2(a), the more time points we use, the less subjects can be used as training subjects. To fully capitalize on the information of all time points and all

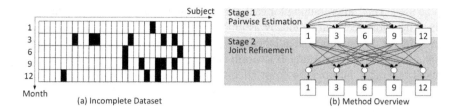

Fig. 2. Overview of our longitudinal infant dataset and the proposed missing data estimation method. In **(a)**, each column indicates a subject, and each row indicates a time point, where the black blocks indicate the missing data at particular time points. In **(b)**, each box with a time-point number stands for the data at the corresponding time point. The directed edges represent the processes of missing data estimation at the target time points (pointed by the arrowhead) by using the data at the available time points (at the tail side). The bidirectional edges in Stage 1 mean that the estimation is performed bidirectionally by exchanging the input time point and the target time point. The circles in Stage 2 mean using multiple time points *jointly*.

subjects, we propose a two-stage method, including (**Stage 1**) pair-wise estimation between different time points to form a pseudo-complete data, and (**Stage 2**) joint refinement based on the pseudo-complete data, as shown in Fig. 2(b).

In **Stage 1**, to capitalize on as many training subjects as possible, the cortical thickness map of a subject at each missing time point is estimated using the data at each of other available time points *independently*, and then these independent estimations are averaged together to obtain an initial estimation. For example, to obtain the initial estimation at 6-months-old, we first use the subjects with available data at both 1- and 6-months-old as training subjects to train a set of decision trees, for estimating the data at 6-months-old based on the data at 1-month-old. Then, after training, for the subjects with available data at 1-month-old but without data at 6-months-old, those trained decision trees are locally assembled as forests to estimate the missing data at 6-months-old. Similarly, we can also obtain the estimation of the missing data at 6-months-old, respectively, based on the available data at each of the 3-, 9-, and 12-months-old. In this way, all available data at all other time points can contribute to the estimation of missing data at 6-months-old. Finally, we average all those estimations (contributed from different time points) as the initial estimation. Similarly, for the missing data at 1-, 3-, 9-, and 12-months-old, the same process can be performed to obtain their initial estimations. After **Stage 1**, all the missing data of all subjects will be approximately recovered, thus providing a pseudo-complete longitudinal dataset.

In **Stage 2**, to take advantage of the longitudinal information and also to make the estimation temporally consistent, the missing data at each time point of each subject is further refined using all the data at all other time points *jointly*. For example, to obtain the final estimation of the missing data at 6-months-old, we use all the subjects that have *real* data at 6-months-old as training subjects to train a set of decision trees, which can estimate the missing data at 6-months-old based on the given data at 1-, 3-, 9-, and 12-months-old jointly. Note that we do not require each training/testing subject to have *real* data at 1-, 3-, 9-, and 12-months-old. If a training/testing subject has missing data at 1-, 3-, 9-, or 12-months-old, its initial estimation that has been estimated in **Stage 1** can be used. Thus, after training for each subject with missing data at 6-months-old, the trained decision trees can be locally assembled as forests to estimate its missing data. Similarly, for the missing data at other time points, the same process can be conducted to obtain their final estimations. It is worth noting that, using the above two stages, our method leverages information from all time points of all subjects for missing data estimation.

3 Results

The dataset we used in the experiments are illustrated in Fig. 2(a), including 31 healthy infants (with 15 infants having missing data), in which each subject was scheduled to be scanned at 1, 3, 6, 9, and 12 months of age. To evaluate our regression model DARF, we conducted an experiment of using cortical thickness and sulcal depth at one time point to estimate cortical thickness at another time point. The motivation to use sulcal depth for helping estimation of cortical thickness is that these two cortical attributes are highly related [18].

To better demonstrate the effectiveness of DARF, we compared it with other three representative methods, including linear regression (LR), global regression forest (GRF), and sparse linear regression (SLR). LR method learned a linear relationship between cortical thickness at a known time point and cortical thickness at missing time point for each vertex on the cortical surface. GRF method trained a single forest for the entire surface, and used spherical location of each vertex as features, in addition to the Haar-like features. SLR is a popular and effective method for high-dimensional data analysis [19, 20]. By setting the coefficients of irrelevant feature elements as zero, SLR is able to extract the most useful features from a high-dimensional feature representation, making it a reasonable competitor of DARF. Specifically, given the target vector $\mathbf{Y} = [y_1, y_2, \ldots, y_n]^T \in \mathbb{R}^n$ and the feature matrix $\mathbf{X} = [\mathbf{X}_1, \mathbf{X}_2, \ldots, \mathbf{X}_n] \in \mathbb{R}^{d \times n}$, SLR method finds the optimal coefficients $\mathbf{A} = [a_1, a_2, \ldots, a_d]^T \in \mathbb{R}^d$ by solving Eq. 2 below, with the constraint that the number of non-zero elements in $\mathbf{A}$ is no more than L.

$$arg\ \min_{\alpha \in \mathbb{R}} \frac{1}{2} \left\| \mathbf{Y} - \mathbf{X}^T \mathbf{A} \right\|_2^2 + \lambda \|\boldsymbol{\alpha}\|_1 \tag{2}$$

To make the comparison fair, we used the same training data with the same features for both SLR and DARF, and we also optimally set $L = 12$ and $\lambda = 0.001$ based on a grid search, which was performed on a subset of the training data.

To quantitatively evaluate the estimation results, we employed two metrics: mean absolute error ($MAE = |\mathbf{T}_e - T_t|/N$) and mean relative error ($MRE = |(\mathbf{T}_e - \mathbf{T}_t)/T_t|/N$), where T_t and T_e are respectively the ground-truth and estimated values of cortical thickness, and N is the number of vertices. Figure 3 provides a comparison of LR, GRF, SLR, and DARF for estimation of vertex-wise cortical thickness map at 9 months of age using cortical attributes at 1 month of age on a representative subject. As we can see, DARF estimated more accurate cortical thickness maps than all the other methods, especially in some highlighted challenging regions, such as the frontal pole, rostral middle frontal gyrus, and supramarginal gyrus.

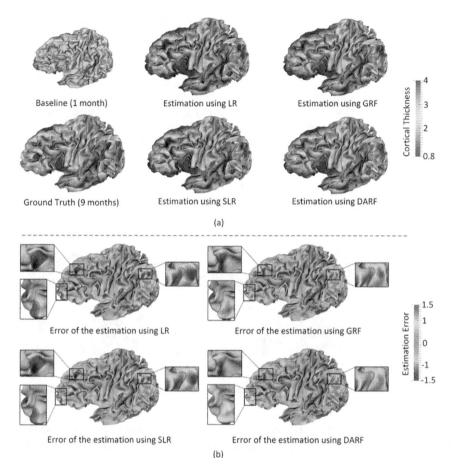

Fig. 3. Estimation of the cortical thickness map at 9 months of age using the data at 1 month of age for a typical infant. (a) shows the cortical thickness maps in mm at 1 and 9 months of age, and the estimation results using different methods, i.e., LR, GRF, SLR, and DARF. (b) shows the vertex-wise error maps in mm by different methods.

For comprehensive comparisons, we repetitively estimated the cortical thickness maps at 3-, 6-, 9-, and 12 months of age using the data at 1 month of age for all the available subjects, and performed a leave-one-out cross validation for each target time point. As reported in Table 1, we can see that according to the estimation accuracy these four methods can be ranked as DARF > SLR > GRF > LR. To statistically demonstrate the advantage of DARF, we also performed paired t-test. Since all the p-values are far less than 0.01, only the p-values of the t-test between DARF and SLR is reported in Table 1. Hence, we can conclude that DARF performs significantly better than the other three methods in estimating vertex-wise cortical thickness maps.

To evaluate the proposed missing data estimation method, we tested our method by recovering the data of cortical thickness at 5 missing time points. Specifically, from our longitudinal dataset (Fig. 2a), we randomly selected 5 subjects that had complete data

Table 1. Quantitative evaluation of the estimation errors of cortical thickness at 3, 6, 9, and 12 months of age, by using different methods, based on the cortical attributes at 1 month of age.

Metric	Methods	3 months	6 months	9 months	12 months
MAE (mm)	LR	0.209 ± 0.033	0.336 ± 0.041	0.342 ± 0.033	0.322 ± 0.028
	GRF	0.209 ± 0.027	0.335 ± 0.039	0340 ± 0.026	0.321 ± 0.025
	SLR	0.207 ± 0.029	0.329 ± 0.040	0.338 ± 0.025	0.320 ± 0.024
	DARF	**0.205 ± 0.027**	**0.316 ± 0.042**	**0.326 ± 0.026**	**0.310 ± 0.026**
	p-value (SLR vs. DARF)	**0.0013**	$\mathbf{3 \times 10^{-13}}$	$\mathbf{1 \times 10^{-9}}$	$\mathbf{4 \times 10^{-9}}$
MRE (%)	LR	10.21 ± 2.03	13.94 ± 1.19	12.95 ± 0.97	12.07 ± 0.72
	GRF	10.17 ± 1.66	13.88 ± 1.21	12.56 ± 0.98	11.87 ± 0.86
	SLR	10.09 ± 1.51	13.12 ± 1.18	12.46 ± 0.97	11.67 ± 0.78
	DARF	**10.00 ± 1.51**	**12.59 ± 1.12**	**12.05 ± 0.93**	**11.30 ± 0.76**
	p-value (SLR vs. DARF)	**0.0032**	$\mathbf{8 \times 10^{-14}}$	$\mathbf{1 \times 10^{-10}}$	$\mathbf{3 \times 10^{-10}}$

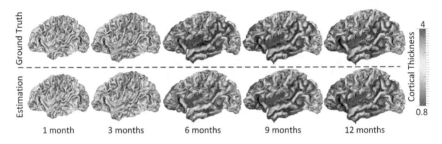

Fig. 4. Estimation of the missing cortical thickness maps (mm) for a typical infant.

at all 5 time points as the reference subjects. For each of these reference subjects, we manually deleted the data at one time point, and then put it back to the dataset. We run our missing data estimation method to recover the missing data, and then compared it with the ground truth. This experiment was repeated 12 times, with each time using 5 different subjects as reference subjects. We also performed paired t-test to statistically compare the results of pairwise estimation (**Stage 1**) and joint refinement (**Stage 2**). Figure 4 shows the results of our method for estimation of cortical thickness at 1, 3, 6, 9, and 12 months of age on a typical infant. The complete quantitative evaluation is reported in Table 2, from which we can conclude that: (1) our method can effectively estimate the missing cortical thickness maps with the average error less than 0.23 mm; and (2) joint refinement significantly improves the results of pairwise estimation. Note that among all time points the estimations were relatively less accurate at around 6 months of age, due to the extremely low image contrast and exceptionally rapid cortex development during this stage [15]. Of note, Table 2 shows better results than Table 1, because only the 1-month-old data was used for estimation in Table 1, while all available time-point data was used in Table 2. We further reported the estimation errors in 35 cortical ROIs, as shown in Fig. 5. We can see that in all ROIs, the joint refinement clearly improves the results, with particularly large improvement in the cingulate cortex, cuneus cortex, orbitofrontal cortex, middle temporal gyrus, pars orbitalis, pericalcarine cortex, and superior frontal gyrus.

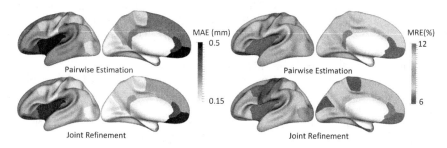

Fig. 5. Errors of estimation of the missing cortical thickness maps at 9 months of age in 35 ROIs.

Table 2. Quantitative evaluation of estimation results for the missing cortical thickness maps using the proposed method.

Target	MAE (mm)			MRE (%)		
	Stage 1	Stage 2	p-value	Stage 1	Stage 2	p-value
1 month	0.179 ± 0.015	**0.169 ± 0.013**	**5 × 10⁻⁴**	8.94 ± 0.89	**8.32 ± 0.65**	**3 × 10⁻⁴**
3 months	0.208 ± 0.027	**0.194 ± 0.025**	**8 × 10⁻⁶**	10.01 ± 1.33	**9.24 ± 1.26**	**6 × 10⁻⁷**
6 months	0.252 ± 0.041	**0.233 ± 0.034**	**2 × 10⁻⁴**	9.91 ± 0.72	**9.08 ± 0.77**	**6 × 10⁻⁶**
9 months	0.261 ± 0.021	**0.225 ± 0.016**	**7 × 10⁻⁸**	9.50 ± 0.56	**8.15 ± 0.50**	**2 × 10⁻⁹**
12 months	0.246 ± 0.019	**0.215 ± 0.016**	**7 × 10⁻¹¹**	9.04 ± 0.46	**7.82 ± 0.49**	**9 × 10⁻¹²**

4 Conclusion

This paper has two major contributions. First, we proposed DARF to ensure the spatial smoothness of regression results and also the computational efficacy, by sharing decision trees with neighboring forests. Second, we proposed a two-stage method to unprecedentedly estimate subject-specific vertex-wise cortical thickness maps at the missing time point(s) in longitudinal infant study, by fully exploiting the available information from all subjects. Of note, our method is very generic and not limited to estimate only cortical thickness, as it can be extended to estimate other cortical anatomical attributes, such as surface area, sulcal depth, and local cortical gyrification [21].

References

1. Gilmore, J.H., Shi, F., Woolson, S.L., Knickmeyer, R.C., Short, S.J., Lin, W., Zhu, H., Hamer, R.M., Styner, M., Shen, D.: Longitudinal development of cortical and subcortical gray matter from birth to 2 years. Cereb. Cortex **22**, 2478–2485 (2012)
2. Li, G., Nie, J., Wang, L., Shi, F., Lin, W., Gilmore, J.H., Shen, D.: Mapping region-specific longitudinal cortical surface expansion from birth to 2 years of age. Cereb. Cortex **23**, 2724–2733 (2013)
3. Li, G., Nie, J., Wang, L., Shi, F., Lyall, A.E., Lin, W., Gilmore, J.H., Shen, D.: Mapping longitudinal hemispheric structural asymmetries of the human cerebral cortex from birth to 2 years of age. Cereb. Cortex **24**, 1289–1300 (2014)

4. Meng, Y., Li, G., Lin, W., Gilmore, J.H., Shen, D.: Spatial distribution and longitudinal development of deep cortical sulcal landmarks in infants. NeuroImage **100**, 206–218 (2014)
5. Nie, J., Li, G., Wang, L., Shi, F., Lin, W., Gilmore, J.H., Shen, D.: Longitudinal development of cortical thickness, folding, and fiber density networks in the first 2 years of life. Hum. Brain Mapp. **35**, 3726–3737 (2014)
6. Awate, S.P., Yushkevich, P.A., Song, Z., Licht, D.J., Gee, J.C.: Cerebral cortical folding analysis with multivariate modeling and testing: studies on gender differences and neonatal development. Neuroimage **53**, 450–459 (2010)
7. Dubois, J., Benders, M., Borradori-Tolsa, C., Cachia, A., Lazeyras, F., Ha-Vinh Leuchter, R., Sizonenko, S.V., Warfield, S.K., Mangin, J.F., Huppi, P.S.: Primary cortical folding in the human newborn: an early marker of later functional development. Brain: J. Neurol. **131**, 2028–2041 (2008)
8. Gilmore, J.H., Lin, W., Prastawa, M.W., Looney, C.B., Vetsa, Y.S., Knickmeyer, R.C., Evans, D.D., Smith, J.K., Hamer, R.M., Lieberman, J.A., Gerig, G.: Regional gray matter growth, sexual dimorphism, and cerebral asymmetry in the neonatal brain. J. Neurosci. Official J. Soc. Neurosci. **27**, 1255–1260 (2007)
9. Schnack, H.G., van Haren, N.E., Brouwer, R.M., Evans, A., Durston, S., Boomsma, D.I., Kahn, R.S., Hulshoff Pol, H.E.: Changes in thickness and surface area of the human cortex and their relationship with intelligence. Cereb. Cortex **25**, 1608–1617 (2015)
10. Lyall, A.E., Shi, F., Geng, X., Woolson, S., Li, G., Wang, L., Hamer, R.M., Shen, D., Gilmore, J.H.: Dynamic development of regional cortical thickness and surface area in early childhood. Cereb. Cortex **25**, 2204–2212 (2015)
11. Troyanskaya, O., Cantor, M., Sherlock, G., Brown, P., Hastie, T., Tibshirani, R., Botstein, D., Altman, R.B.: Missing value estimation methods for DNA microarrays. Bioinformatics **17**, 520–525 (2001)
12. Tsiporkova, E., Boeva, V.: Two-pass imputation algorithm for missing value estimation in gene expression time series. J. Bioinf. Comput. Biol. **5**, 1005–1022 (2007)
13. Candès, E., Recht, B.: Exact matrix completion via convex optimization. Found. Comput. Math. **9**, 717–772 (2009)
14. Liu, J., Musialski, P., Wonka, P., Ye, J.: Tensor completion for estimating missing values in visual data. IEEE Trans. Pattern Anal. Mach. Intell. **35**, 208–220 (2013)
15. Li, G., Nie, J., Wang, L., Shi, F., Gilmore, J.H., Lin, W., Shen, D.: Measuring the dynamic longitudinal cortex development in infants by reconstruction of temporally consistent cortical surfaces. Neuroimage **90**, 266–279 (2014)
16. Li, G., Wang, L., Shi, F., Lin, W., Shen, D.: Constructing 4D infant cortical surface atlases based on dynamic developmental trajectories of the cortex. Med. Image Comput. Comput. Assist. Interv. **17**, 89–96 (2014)
17. Breiman, L.: Random forests. Mach. Learn. **45**, 5–32 (2001)
18. Fischl, B., Dale, A.M.: Measuring the thickness of the human cerebral cortex from magnetic resonance images. Proc. Natl. Acad. Sci. USA **97**, 11050–11055 (2000)
19. Tibshirani, R.: Regression shrinkage and selection via the Lasso. J. R. Stat. Soc. B (Methodological) **58**, 267–288 (1996)
20. Zhang, S., Zhan, Y., Dewan, M., Huang, J., Metaxas, D.N., Zhou, X.S.: Towards robust and effective shape modeling: sparse shape composition. Med. Image Anal. **16**, 265–277 (2012)
21. Li, G., Wang, L., Shi, F., Lyall, A.E., Lin, W., Gilmore, J.H., Shen, D.: Mapping longitudinal development of local cortical gyrification in infants from birth to 2 years of age. J. Neurosci. **34**, 4228–4238 (2014)

Advanced Methods for Image Analysis

Calibrationless Parallel Dynamic MRI with Joint Temporal Sparsity

Yang Yu[1]([✉]), Zhennan Yan[1], Li Feng[2], Dimitris Metaxas[1], and Leon Axel[2]

[1] Department of Computer Science, Rutgers University, Piscataway, NJ, USA
yyu@cs.rutgers.edu
[2] Department of Medicine, New York University, New York, NY, USA

Abstract. In this paper, we propose a novel calibrationless method for parallel dynamic magnetic resonance imaging (MRI) reconstruction, which overcomes the limitations posed by traditional MRI reconstruction methods that require accurate coil calibration. Thus, calibrationless methods, which remove the requirement of coil sensitivity profiles for MRI reconstruction, are suitable for dynamic MRI. Dynamic MRI contains rich temporal redundant information, i.e., the pixel intensities change smoothly over time. This property can be modeled as various types of temporal sparse priors, in the Fourier transform domain, or in the image domain using finite differences. In addition, the temporally changing patterns of pixels are similar in the various coils, since their signals are different due to the coil sensitivity profiles. Therefore, we model the parallel dynamic MRI problems as joint temporal sparsity tasks, and develop a class of algorithms to solve them efficiently. Experiments on parallel dynamic MRI datasets demonstrate that our proposed methods outperform the state-of-the-art parallel MRI reconstruction algorithms.

1 Introduction

Multi-coil parallel magnetic resonance imaging (MRI) is a powerful technique introduced [16] to accelerate the image acquisition. The image signals from a patient are simultaneously collected by a group of spatially distributed coils with different sensitivity profiles. Each coil, instead of sampling the full k-space, only samples it partially. Since less sampling is required for each coil, the time of the MRI scanning is reduced by parallel imaging without compromising the quality. The MRI image is then reconstructed by combining the information from all the coils based on their sensitivity profiles. In parallel MRI, it is an ill-posed problem to reconstruct both the MRI image and the coil sensitivity maps jointly. Therefore, parallel MRI reconstruction methods, e.g., SMASH [16] and SENSE [14], require estimation of the coil sensitivity profiles before image reconstruction. These methods often proceed in two stages: (1) the calibration stage, in which the sensitivity profiles are explicitly estimated; (2) the reconstruction stage, in which the image is reconstructed based on the estimated sensitivity maps. A major limitation is that the reconstruction accuracy is sensitive to the calibration accuracy.

© Springer International Publishing Switzerland 2016
B. Menze et al. (Eds.): MCV Workshop 2015, LNCS 9601, pp. 95–102, 2016.
DOI: 10.1007/978-3-319-42016-5_9

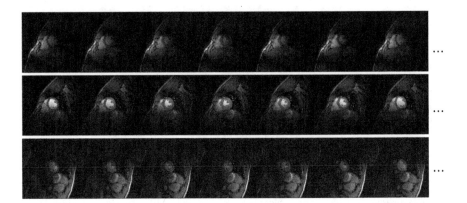

Fig. 1. Sensitivity encoded images from different coils (rows) and frames (columns).

In dynamic multi-coil parallel MRI, the cost of the calibration is amplified, since the sensitivity profiles of all coils change due to the patient's movements. Previous work [3,12,13] used SENSE [14] to reconstruct the parallel dynamic MRI images, where the explicit coil sensitivity estimations are required at each time frame. This does not only increase the acquisition time, but may also introduce calibration errors due to the patient's movements. In cardiac MRI, patients are required to hold their breath in each scan. The time of the breath holding is only tens of second for normal people, so the calibration and reconstruction scans may be acquired in different respiratory periods. However, the patients may hold their breath at different position each time. The varying displacement of the chest will cause a misalignment between the scans during the calibration and reconstruction stages. Such movement-caused inconsistencies in the coil sensitivity estimation may result in significant visual artifacts in reconstructed images [4].

To avoid the calibration step for parallel MRI, some calibrationless methods [5,11,15] have been proposed recently. Instead of reconstructing the original image directly, they reconstruct the sensitivity encoded images for all the coils. The different coils focus on the same anatomical cross-section during the scan. They produce different images only due to their different sensitivity profiles. Figure 1 shows some sample sensitivity encoded images from different coils. Different regions are highlighted due to the coil sensitivity profiles, while the intrinsic image information remains the same. Therefore, all the sensitivity encoded images should have high valued responses to sparsifying transforms at the same positions. Majumdar and Ward [11] reconstructed the parallel MRI images based on the fact that the position of the high valued wavelet transform coefficients in different sensitivity encoded coil images remain the same. They applied a group sparse constraint to the wavelet transform coefficients for all the images, and solved the optimization problem with Majorization-Minimization. Chen et al. [5] utilized the spatial total variation as the image constraint, and the images from different coils are reconstructed based on joint total variation. Shin et al. [15]

explored the low rank property of the image blocks in the k-space data, and optimized a structured low-rank matrix completion problem to generate coil-by-coil sensitivity encoded images.

In this work, we propose a new parallel MRI method for dynamic images, called calibrationless dynamic MRI with joint temporal sparsity. Our method is an extension of the temporal sparse SENSE method [13], which explores the benefit of temporal sparse properties of the MRI sequence. The sparse property has already been extensively used for MR image reconstruction [13], segmentation [18], and motion tracking [17]. We further extend the sparse method with group structure constraints. Unlike previous calibrationless methods, we do not assume any spatial sparse constraints. The temporal signal contains more redundancy, due to the smoothness of the displacement field. In addition, the signals among different coils are different, due to their sensitivity profiles. Due to the smoothness of the coil sensitivity maps, the temporal changing patterns of intensities in the various coil images are similar. Therefore, we utilize the smoothness of the temporal changes and the correlation of the coil images to propose a joint temporal sparse model to reconstruct parallel dynamic images simultaneously. We present two variants using different temporal sparsifying operators. They are compared to the state-of-the-art parallel dynamic MRI reconstruction algorithms, and both show improved performance.

2   Method

In this section, we first introduce the dynamic MRI reconstruction based on compressed sensing and SENSE [13]. Then we present our calibrationless method, which reconstructs the image without the coil sensitivity profiles. Finally, the optimization algorithms are discussed for two typical temporal sparse constraints in our framework.

2.1   k-t SPARSE-SENSE

The MRI reconstruction techniques have attracted increasing attention in recent years, due to improved results based on compressed sensing [7,9]. The key idea for compressed sensing in MRI, is to explore the resulting image compressibility due to the image sparseness under certain transforms, e.g., wavelet. By enforcing these sparse priors, less sampling is required to acquire and reconstruct the MRI image, which is almost lossless. Compressed sensing is suitable for dynamic MRI since there is redundant information in the sequential temporal data. This is very similar to video compression, where the inter-frame encoding is much more efficient than the intra-frame encoding. For example, in k-t SPARSE-SENSE [13], a temporal Fourier transform is used to sparsify the MRI image sequence.

Let $\bar{X} \in \mathbb{R}^{M \times N \times T}$ denote a dynamic MRI image sequence, where the image size is $M \times N$, and the number of frames is T. Assuming there are C parallel coils used in the imaging process, under-sampled k-space data y_{ct} are acquired from coil $c \in \{1, ..., C\}$ at time $t \in \{1, ..., T\}$. The problem of reconstructing $\bar{X}$ is formulated as:

$$\underset{\bar{X}}{\mathrm{argmin}}\{\frac{1}{2}\sum_{c=1}^{C}\sum_{t=1}^{T}\|F_{ct}S_{ct}\bar{X}_t - y_{ct}\|_2^2 + \lambda\sum_{i=1}^{M}\sum_{j=1}^{N}\|\Phi\bar{X}_{ij}\|_1\} \tag{1}$$

where F_{ct} is the partial Fourier transform, Φ is a temporal sparsifying operator on each pixel (e.g., temporal Fourier transform), and λ is the sparsity parameter. Before solving Eq. (1), the coil sensitivity profiles S_{ct} are estimated in the calibration stage.

2.2   Our Approach: Joint Temporal Sparsity

In this paper, we present a calibrationless method to reconstruct the image without coil sensitivity estimation. Since the signals on all the coils are acquired from the same anatomical cross section, they are closely correlated with each other. The signals have similar sparse properties for all the coils, i.e., the corresponding transform terms are likely to be zeros or not at the same time. Therefore, we propose joint temporal sparse priors for dynamic MRI reconstruction, to implicitly enforce the relations among different coils. The coil sensitivity profiles are not required for our method, which eliminates a significant source of error in the reconstructed MRI images.

The coil-dependent sensitivity-encoded dynamic images $X \in \mathbb{R}^{M \times N \times T \times C}$ are reconstructed in our proposed calibrationless algorithm, instead of the final image $\bar{X}$. The reason is that each sensitivity-encoded image $X_{ct} = S_{ct}\bar{X}_t$ contains its coil sensitivity profile in itself, and therefore the S_{ct} is not required to be estimated explicitly to solve the reconstruction. In our approach, the problem of reconstructing the sensitivity-encoded images X based on the MRI signals y_{ct} is formulated as:

$$\underset{X}{\mathrm{argmin}}\{\frac{1}{2}\sum_{c=1}^{C}\sum_{t=1}^{T}\|F_{ct}X_{ct} - y_{ct}\|_2^2 + \lambda\sum_{i=1}^{M}\sum_{j=1}^{N}\|\Phi X_{ij}\|_{2,1}\} \tag{2}$$

where $\|\cdot\|_{2,1}$ is the $L2,1$ norm, which regularizes the pixel-by-pixel temporal sparseness jointly among coils. Let $Z_{ij} = \Phi X_{ij}$ be the transformed image data at one pixel location for all C coils and T frames. The size of matrix Z_{ij} is $B \times C$, where B is the dimensionality of the transform Φ, e.g., the number of coefficients in the temporal Fourier transform. The $L2,1$ norm can be rewritten as:

$$\|Z_{ij}\|_{2,1} = \sum_{b=1}^{B}\|Z_{ijb}\|_2 = \sum_{b=1}^{B}\left(\sum_{c=1}^{C}|Z_{ijcb}|^2\right)^{\frac{1}{2}} \tag{3}$$

where the column-wise $L2$ norm is first applied to the coil dimension of Z_{ij}, and then the row-wise $L1$ norm is applied to the transform's dimension. In this way, the corresponding terms in different coils are likely to be zero or not at the same time. Various types of sparsifying operators can be used for temporal MRI image reconstruction since, as we mentioned, the pixel variation over time is smooth. Typical choices include the temporal Fourier transform and temporal finite differences.

Although the coil sensitivity profiles are removed from the formulation, the coil images are still correlated with each other, based on joint sparse constraints. Finally, since these are sensitivity-encoded images they are combined via a sum of squares approach [6,10] to produce the final image.

2.3 Algorithm

There are generally two types of joint sparse priors that can be used, based on whether the inverse transform is available. The problem is relatively easy when there is an invertible transform like the temporal Fourier transform, since $X_{ij} = \Phi_F^T Z_{ij}$ can be represented as a function of Z. Therefore, we rewrite Eq. 2 using the Fourier transform to solve for Z:

$$\underset{Z}{\operatorname{argmin}}\{\frac{1}{2}\sum_{c=1}^{C}\|F_c\Phi_F^T Z_c - y_c\|_2^2 + \lambda\sum_{i=1}^{M}\sum_{j=1}^{N}\|Z_{ij}\|_{2,1}\} \tag{4}$$

This formulation can be directly solved with FISTA [2] which requires solving the following subproblem for all pixels in each iteration:

$$\underset{Z_{ij}}{\operatorname{argmin}}\{\frac{1}{2}\|Z_{ij} - \tilde{Z}_{ij}\|_2^2 + \lambda\|Z_{ij}\|_{2,1}\} \tag{5}$$

where $\tilde{Z}_{ij}$ is known at the beginning of the iteration. This subproblem has the following analytical solution:

$$Z_{ijt} = \begin{cases} \frac{\|Z_{ijt}\|_2 - \lambda}{\|Z_{ijt}\|_2} Z_{ijt} & \text{if } \|Z_{ijt}\|_2 > \lambda \\ 0 & \text{otherwise} \end{cases} \tag{6}$$

The problem is more complex when no invertible transform exists, like the finite differences. We still use FISTA to solve the problem, while the subproblem is more complex:

$$\underset{X_{ij}}{\operatorname{argmin}}\{\frac{1}{2}\|X_{ij} - \tilde{X}_{ij}\|_2^2 + \lambda\|\Phi_D X_{ij}\|_{2,1}\} \tag{7}$$

where $\tilde{X}$ is known for each iteration. Following previous work [1,8], we consider the dual problem for Eq. 7. Let $P \in \mathbb{R}^{C\times(T-1)}$, which satisfies:

$$\sum_{c=1}^{C} P_{ct}^2 \le 1 \quad \forall t, \quad |P_{ct}| \le 1 \quad \forall c,t \tag{8}$$

The relation between X and P is defined by a linear operator $\mathcal{L}(P)_{ct} = P_{ct} - P_{c(t-1)}$ and the corresponding inverse operator $\mathcal{L}^T(X) = P$, where $P_{ct} = X_{ct} - X_{ct+1}$. The optimal solution for Eq. 7 is $X = \tilde{X} - \lambda\mathcal{L}(P^*)$, based on [1], where P^* is the optimal solution for the dual problem $\min_P \frac{1}{2}\|\tilde{X} - \lambda\mathcal{L}(P)\|_2^2$. This dual problem can also be solved by FISTA iteratively.

3   Experiments

The experiments were conducted on the cardiac parallel dynamic MRI dataset. The cardiac cine MRI recorded the heart motion during a cardiac cycle for assessment of its function. A Steady State Free Precession (SSFP) pulse sequence with cartesian sampling was employed for data acquisition on a 1.5T Siemens scanner equipped with the standard 32-element matrix coil array.

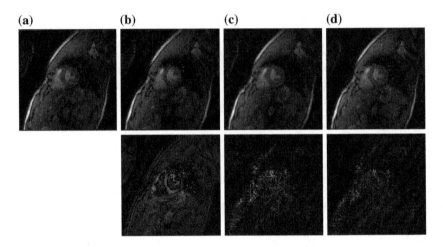

Fig. 2. The visual results of different methods. (a) The ground truth image, (b) k-t SPARSE SENSE, (c) Our proposed method with Fourier transform, and (d) Our proposed method with finite differences. The second row are the error images of these methods.

We first compare our proposed joint temporal sparse method with k-t SPARSE-SENSE [13], which is a calibration based method. Uniform random sampling masks were used with reduction factor four to under-sample the original k-space data. Figure 2 shows the reconstruction results at the end of systole. Two types of temporal constraints, Fourier transform and finite differences, are validated in our framework. Both variants of our methods show similar visual results as k-t SPARSE-SENSE. This shows the benefit of the joint sparseness prior for temporal signals. Notice that the coil sensitivity maps, which were provided for k-t SPARSE-SENSE during the reconstruction, are unknown to our methods.

We then compared our proposed method to other calibrationless algorithms quantitatively, including k-t SPARSE-SENSE (publicly available code exists), CaLM MRI [11], and Joint Total Variation [5] (based on our own implementations). Since CaLM MRI and Joint Total Variation were designed for static MR image reconstruction, we simply applied their methods to our dynamic MR images frame by frame. To reduce randomness, we ran each algorithm 10 times to obtain the average results. Table 1 shows the average SNRs and computing

Table 1. Comparison of Signal-to-Noise Ratio (SNR) and computing times of different calibrationless MRI reconstruction methods

Method	SNR (dB)	Time (s)
k-t SPARSE-SENSE [13]	22.1	362.2
CaLM MRI [11]	17.8	624.5
Joint Total Variation [5]	19.8	497.0
Proposed with Fourier transform	24.5	**160.7**
Proposed with finite differences	**26.6**	281.9

times for all the methods. The two variants of our proposed method showed consistently better performance than all the other calibrationless algorithms, due to our novel approach, which is based on the temporal sparse priors. CaLM MRI [11] and joint total variation [5] are slower than our temporal sparse constraint approach, since the 2D spatial constraints have higher computing cost. Although k-t SPARSE-SENSE utilized additional coil sensitivity information, it is still slower than our proposed algorithms due to the inefficient optimization algorithm. Our method does not require coil calibration. It leads to further reductions in the time and the motion errors in dynamic MRI acquisitions.

4   Conclusions

We have proposed a novel calibrationless algorithm to accelerate the dynamic MRI reconstructions with parallel imaging and compressed sensing. The main novelty is in the use of a joint temporal sparsity approach, which does not require one to estimate the coil calibration. The temporal sparse priors are utilized in a joint way to exploit both signal sparseness and coil correlation. Two typical temporal sparse priors, the Fourier transform and the finite differences, were validated with our proposed joint sparse optimization algorithms. The experiments show that the proposed method outperforms the state-of-art parallel dynamic MRI reconstruction algorithms. In addition, the proposed method is better than other calibrationless algorithms in terms of both accuracy and efficiency and has the potential to improve the efficiency of clinical MRI.

Acknowledgments. The research is partially supported by the grant NIH 1R01HL127661-01.

References

1. Beck, A., Teboulle, M.: Fast gradient-based algorithms for constrained total variation image denoising and deblurring problems. IEEE Trans. Image Process. **18**(11), 2419–2434 (2009)
2. Beck, A., Teboulle, M.: A fast iterative shrinkage-thresholding algorithm for linear inverse problems. SIAM J. Imaging Sci. **2**(1), 183–202 (2009)

3. Bilen, C., Wang, Y., Selesnick, I.: High-speed compressed sensing reconstruction in dynamic parallel MRI using augmented lagrangian and parallel processing. IEEE J. Emerg. Sel. Top. Circuits Syst. **2**(3), 370–379 (2012)
4. Blaimer, M., Breuer, F., Mueller, M., Heidemann, R.M., Griswold, M.A., Jakob, P.M.: SMASH, SENSE, PILS, GRAPPA: how to choose the optimal method. Top. Magn. Reson. Imaging **15**(4), 223–236 (2004)
5. Chen, C., Li, Y., Huang, J.: Calibrationless parallel MRI with joint total variation regularization. In: Mori, K., Sakuma, I., Sato, Y., Barillot, C., Navab, N. (eds.) MICCAI 2013, Part III. LNCS, vol. 8151, pp. 106–114. Springer, Heidelberg (2013)
6. Griswold, M.A., Jakob, P.M., Heidemann, R.M., Nittka, M., Jellus, V., Wang, J., Kiefer, B., Haase, A.: Generalized autocalibrating partially parallel acquisitions (GRAPPA). Magn. Reson. Med. **47**(6), 1202–1210 (2002)
7. Huang, J., Zhang, S., Metaxas, D.: Efficient MR image reconstruction for compressed MR imaging. Med. Image Anal. **15**(5), 670–679 (2011). Special Issue on the 2010 Conference on Medical Image Computing and Computer-Assisted Intervention
8. Liu, J., Yuan, L., Ye, J.: An efficient algorithm for a class of fused lasso problems. In: Proceedings of the 16th ACM SIGKDD International Conference on Knowledge Discovery and Data Mining, pp. 323–332. ACM, New York (2010)
9. Lustig, M., Donoho, D., Pauly, J.M.: Sparse MRI: the application of compressed sensing for rapid MR imaging. Magn. Reson. Med. **58**(6), 1182–1195 (2007)
10. Lustig, M., Pauly, J.M.: SPIRiT: iterative self-consistent parallel imaging reconstruction from arbitrary k-space. Magn. Reson. Med. **64**(2), 457–471 (2010)
11. Majumdar, A., Ward, R.K.: Calibration-less multi-coil MR image reconstruction. Magn. Reson. Imaging **30**(7), 1032–1045 (2012)
12. Otazo, R., Feng, L., Chandarana, H., Block, T., Axel, L., Sodickson, D.: Combination of compressed sensing and parallel imaging for highly-accelerated dynamic MRI. In: 9th IEEE International Symposium on Biomedical Imaging, pp. 980–983 (2012)
13. Otazo, R., Kim, D., Axel, L., Sodickson, D.K.: Combination of compressed sensing and parallel imaging for highly accelerated first-pass cardiac perfusion MRI. Magn. Reson. Med. **64**(3), 767–776 (2010)
14. Pruessmann, K.P., Weiger, M., Scheidegger, M.B., Boesiger, P.: Sense: sensitivity encoding for fast MRI. Magn. Reson. Med. **42**(5), 952–962 (1999)
15. Shin, P.J., Larson, P.E.Z., Ohliger, M.A., Elad, M., Pauly, J.M., Vigneron, D.B., Lustig, M.: Calibrationless parallel imaging reconstruction based on structured low-rank matrix completion. Magn. Reson. Med. **72**(4), 959–970 (2014)
16. Sodickson, D.K., Manning, W.J.: Simultaneous acquisition of spatial harmonics (SMASH): fast imaging with radiofrequency coil arrays. Magn. Reson. Med. **38**(4), 591–603 (1997)
17. Yu, Y., Zhang, S., Li, K., Metaxas, D., Axel, L.: Deformable models with sparsity constraints for cardiac motion analysis. Med. Image Anal. **18**(6), 927–937 (2014). Sparse Methods for Signal Reconstruction and Medical Image Analysis
18. Zhang, S., Zhan, Y., Dewan, M., Huang, J., Metaxas, D.N., Zhou, X.S.: Towards robust and effective shape modeling: sparse shape composition. Med. Image Anal. **16**(1), 265–277 (2012)

Creating a Large-Scale Silver Corpus from Multiple Algorithmic Segmentations

Markus Krenn[1]([⊠]), Matthias Dorfer[2], Oscar Alfonso Jiménez del Toro[3],
Henning Müller[3], Bjoern Menze[4], Marc-André Weber[5], Allan Hanbury[6],
and Georg Langs[1]

[1] Computational Imaging Research (CIR) Lab, Department of Biomedical Imaging
and Image-guided Therapy, Medical University of Vienna, Vienna, Austria
`markus.krenn@meduniwien.ac.at`
[2] Department of Computational Perception,
Johannes Kepler University (JKU), Linz, Austria
[3] University of Applied Sciences Western Switzerland (HES-SO), Sierre, Switzerland
[4] Institute for Advanced Study and Department of Computer Science,
Technische Universität München, Munich, Germany
[5] Department of Diagnostic and Interventional Radiology,
University of Heidelberg, Heidelberg, Germany
[6] Institute of Software Technology and Interactive Systems,
TU Wien, Vienna, Austria

Abstract. Currently, increasingly large medical imaging data sets
become available for research and are analysed by a range of algorithms
segmenting anatomical structures automatically and interactively. While
they provide segmentations on a much larger scale than possible to
achieve with expert annotators, they are typically less accurate than
experts. We present and compare approaches to estimate segmentations
on large imaging data sets based on a small number of expert annotated examples, and algorithmic segmentations on a much larger data
set. Results demonstrate that combining algorithmic segmentations is
reliably outperforming the average individual algorithm. Furthermore,
injecting organ specific reliability assessments of algorithms based on
expert annotations improves accuracy compared to standard label fusion
algorithms. The proposed methods are particularly relevant in putting
the results of large image analysis algorithm benchmarks to long-term
use.

Keywords: Segmentation · Label fusion · Silver corpus

1 Introduction

Annotations are an important basis when developing algorithms that segment
anatomical structures in medical imaging data. For relatively small sets, they
can be manually generated by experts, and serve as means for the training, and
evaluation of algorithms. If multiple annotations are available for the same target, label fusion algorithms such as STAPLE [26] provide improved estimates for

© Springer International Publishing Switzerland 2016
B. Menze et al. (Eds.): MCV Workshop 2015, LNCS 9601, pp. 103–115, 2016.
DOI: 10.1007/978-3-319-42016-5_10

true segmentations. Recently, increasingly large data sets have become available to the research community [11]. Such datasets are often part of challenges, where a large number of state of the art algorithms are applied to localize or segment anatomical structures. In this paper we propose and compare approaches to estimate true segmentations on large medical imaging data, if expert annotations are available for only a small sub-set and less reliable algorithmic annotations are available for all data.

Label fusion approaches in medical image segmentation aim at finding the true (hidden) segmentation of a structure in an image by estimating a *consensus* of multiple segmentation estimates. Independent noise in different annotations causes the consensus to correct this variability and yield significantly more accurate segmentations than those derived from a single source [18,22]. For instance, *majority voting* assigns the label with most *votes* among annotators to each voxel [8,15,16]. In the context of multi-atlas label fusion additional weighting or *weighted voting* based on image similarity can further improve results [2]. Further improvement can be gained by fusing labels of a well chosen sub-set of atlases [1] Fusing multiple atlas segmentations significantly outperforms single atlas segmentations [21]. One downside of weighting schemes, is that image similarity is a limited predictor of registration accuracy [2,18]. Therefore, a range of approaches takes multiple annotations into account to assess consistency as a basis for estimating their reliability. Label fusion via *Simultaneous Truth And Performance Level Estimation (STAPLE)* [26] estimates performances and weights of contributing segmentations based on an expectation maximization. STAPLE simultaneously computes performance estimates based on sensitivity and specificity of contributing segmentations during maximization and establishes an estimate of the hidden ground truth segmentation, given performance estimates in the expectation step [26]. It outperforms majority voting, and competes with weighted voting approaches [1]. A *Selective and Iterative Method for Performance Level Estimation (SIMPLE)* proposed in [18] is another iterative label fusion algorithm. Similar to STAPLE it simultaneously computes an estimate of the hidden true segmentation and estimates performances of each contributing segmentation. SIMPLE additionally discards poorly performing segmentations during the fusion process and computes segmentation performances based on a spatial overlap measure of involved segmentations to the current estimate of the hidden ground true segmentation. In case of fusing a small number of expert annotations SIMPLE and STAPLE are reported to perform equally [18].

While these insights are important, existing approaches assume that we face a set of annotators with initially equal competency estimates. In this paper we extend these approaches to cases, where we have a small set of high-quality, or 'expert' annotations (gold corpus), and a large set of algorithmic and possibly less accurate annotations. We show how to use this for estimating segmentations of anatomical structures on a large data set, resulting in a so-called *silver corpus*.

We calculate a silver corpus annotation of anatomical structures in medical images by fusing gold corpus annotations from a limited number of templates by multi-atlas label fusion, and additional algorithmic estimates of the annotations.

CT	CTce	MRT1	MRT1cefs

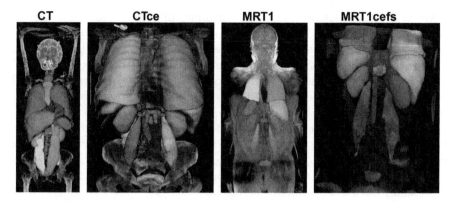

Fig. 1. Illustrations of generated silver corpus annotations of one volume in each modality. Volumes and annotations will be publicly available for the research community.

We estimate the reliability of each algorithm and corresponding weights based on gold corpus annotations on a limited number of cases.

We evaluate different strategies of fusing algorithmic segmentations, and estimate their reliability either by consensus, or by comparison across the annotation sets (gold corpus and algorithmic). Finally we demonstrate that the proposed approach consistently outperforms the average algorithm. Injecting reliability estimates further improves accuracy. We detail the benefit of specific fusion strategies, and provide a comprehensive evaluation of all approaches on 20 anatomical structures in 40 volumes of four different modalities.

We finally apply the best performing fusion method to 264 cases of the evaluated modalities that were part of the VISCERAL challenges [19]. We make the resulting silver corpus that contains 4323 annotated anatomical structures available for the research community. Visualizations of generated silver corpus annotations of one volume of each evaluated modality are shown in Fig. 1.

2   Method

We start with a formal definition of our problem setting. Then, we explain the algorithm for silver corpus label fusion from expert annotations on a small set of cases, and multiple algorithmic annotations for each case. To facilitate reading we explain the segmentation of one anatomical structure in one target image of the silver corpus. This generalizes to arbitrary structures since organs, and target images are treated independently in the proposed approach.

2.1   Problem Setting

Given a segmentation gold corpus as the set of N expert annotated atlases $\mathfrak{A} = \langle \mathbf{I}_1, \ldots, \mathbf{I}_N; \mathbf{L}_1, \ldots, \mathbf{L}_N \rangle$ where an atlas $(\mathbf{I}_n, \mathbf{L}_n)$ is defined as a tuple, containing image $\mathbf{I}_n$ and binary label image (annotation) $\mathbf{L}_n$. We aim to compute a silver standard annotation $\mathbf{L}_T'$ for each organ in a target image (image or volume) $\mathbf{I}_T$ by fusing data that is typically available during benchmarks or competitions. Benchmark data addresses the scenario where the gold corpus $\mathfrak{A}$ is complemented by a set of P automatic segmentation estimates $\mathcal{P} = \langle \hat{\mathbf{L}}_T^1, \dots \hat{\mathbf{L}}_T^P \rangle$ obtained by algorithms that are applied to target image $\mathbf{I}_T$. Each binary label image $\hat{\mathbf{L}}_T^p$ holds the segmentation estimate of algorithm p in target image $\mathbf{I}_T$. The atlas annotations are non-linearly mapped to $\mathbf{I}_T$ using image registration. We compute transformations $T_n(\mathbf{x})$ so that $\mathbf{I}_T(\mathbf{x}) \sim \mathbf{I}_n(T_n(\mathbf{x}))$ and transfer the corresponding annotations $\mathbf{L}_n$ towards the target volume, by applying the same transformation $\tilde{\mathbf{L}}_n(\mathbf{x}) = \mathbf{L}_n(T_n(\mathbf{x}))$. Our goal is to compute a segmentation silver corpus by introducing a label fusion approach taking both, gold corpus $\mathfrak{A}$ as well as algorithmic label estimates $\mathcal{P}$ into account.

2.2   Atlas Registration and Selection

We first map atlas annotations $\mathbf{L}_n$ to the target image in a two step procedure. Inspired by [1] we first evaluate the *Normalized Mutual Information* (NMI) for each pair of an atlas image $\mathbf{I}_n$ and the target image $\mathbf{I}_T$ [24].

After ranking all atlases based on their NMI to $\mathbf{I}_T$, the framework selects the set of top ranked J atlases and computes segmentation estimates of the desired structure in $\mathbf{I}_T$ for each selected atlas by a two step registration process: **1. Registration:** A non-linear alignment between $\mathbf{I}_T$ and each atlas image $\mathbf{I}_n$ is established (for details see Sect. 3), resulting in a transformation T_n, that maps $\mathbf{I}_T$ to $\mathbf{I}_n$ so that $\mathbf{I}_T(x) \approx \mathbf{I}_n(T_n(x))$. **2. Label propagation:** The computed transformation is used to compute a segmentation estimation of atlas n in the target image, denoted as $\tilde{\mathbf{L}}_T(x) = \mathbf{L}_n(T_n(x))$. We denote the set of J atlas based labelings of the target image $\mathbf{I}_T$ as $\mathcal{A} = \langle \tilde{\mathbf{L}}_1, \dots, \tilde{\mathbf{L}}_J \rangle$.

2.3   Computing Weights of Segmentation Estimates

The previous steps result in two sets of labelings for the target image: mapped gold corpus atlas annotations $\mathcal{A}$ and annotations by algorithms $\mathcal{P}$. Inspired by the work in [2], we perform weighted label fusion to generate $\mathbf{L}_T'$. In the following we explain how to determine the weights of individual segmentations.

Obtaining Atlas Weights. We derive atlas segmentation performance estimates by leave-one-out cross validation on the test set. We propagate each annotation $\mathbf{L}_n$ to all remaining atlases based on non-rigid pair-wise registration of the corresponding images. We evaluate the overlap of propagated annotations by comparing them to the native expert annotation in the atlas image using the Dice coefficient [3]. The weight v_n of an atlas annotator $\tilde{\mathbf{L}}_n$ is the average Dice [3] coefficient of its segmentations propagated to all other atlas images, and the corresponding expert annotation. This results in weights $\mathbf{v} = v_1, \dots v_N$.

Obtaining Algorithm Weights. To derive performance estimates $\mathbf{w} = w_1, \ldots w_P$ of the algorithms, each algorithm is applied to all test set atlas volumes. Similar to atlas weights, the weights are calculated by averaging the Dice coefficients [3] of computed segmentations and atlas annotations.

2.4   Fusion

As final step we fuse propagated atlas segmentations $\mathcal{A}$ and algorithmic segmentations $\mathcal{P}$ to the resulting silver corpus annotation $\mathbf{L}'_T$ for the targeted structure. In the following we explain four label fusion approaches and compare them in the experiment section. After calculating weights of atlas- and algorithm annotations individually, we treat them equally during fusion, we denote $\mathcal{L} = \langle \mathbf{L}_1, \ldots, \mathbf{L}_M \rangle$ as a set of M binary label images and $\mathbf{u} = u_1, \ldots u_M$ as a vector of corresponding segmentation weights. $\mathbf{L}'_T(\mathbf{x})$ is the final segmentation estimate in $\mathbf{I}_T$.

1. **Majority Vote (MV):** The computed segmentation performance estimates are not considered during fusion and all contributing segmentations are weighted equally. Each voxel $\mathbf{x}$ of $\mathbf{L}'_T$ is assigned with the label that is most frequent in corresponding voxels of all contributing segmentation estimates:

$$\mathbf{L}'_T(\mathbf{x}) = \begin{cases} 1, & \left(\sum_{i=1}^{M} \mathbf{L}_i(\mathbf{x}) \right) \geq \frac{M}{2} \\ 0, & \left(\sum_{i=1}^{M} \mathbf{L}_i(\mathbf{x}) \right) < \frac{M}{2} \end{cases} \quad (1)$$

2. **Organ Level Weighted Voting:** $\mathbf{L}'_T$ is derived by a majority vote where the impact of each $\mathbf{L}_i \in \mathcal{L}$ is weighted by u_i. Since weights are determined for each organ independently, we call this algorithm Organ Level Weighted Voting (OLWV).

$$\mathbf{L}'_T(\mathbf{x}) = \begin{cases} 1, & \left(\sum_{i=1}^{M} \mathbf{L}_i(\mathbf{x}) \cdot u_i \right) \geq \frac{\sum u}{2} \\ 0, & \left(\sum_{i=1}^{M} \mathbf{L}_i(\mathbf{x}) \cdot u_i \right) < \frac{\sum u}{2} \end{cases} \quad (2)$$

3. **STAPLE:** For evaluation in this work we use the binary version of the STAPLE algorithm [26]. STAPLE takes a set of binary label images $\mathcal{L}$ as input and computes an estimation of the hidden ground truth $\mathbf{L}'_T$ based on expectation maximization [26]. We refer to STAPLE segmentations as $\mathbf{L}'_T = STAPLE(\mathcal{L})$.
4. **SIMPLE:** An implementation of SIMPLE as proposed in [18] is used in our work. Besides $\mathcal{L}$, the algorithm is parametrized by k and α, where α influences the performance level that contributing segmentations must exceed to remain in the set of contributing segmentation and k defines the number of iterations in which segmentations are kept for fusion even though the performance threshold is not reached. Optional, SIMPLE takes initial segmentation weights into account. We refer to SIMPLE segmentations computed without initialization as $\mathbf{L}'_T = SIMPLE(\mathcal{L}, k, \alpha)$ and as $\mathbf{L}'_T = SIMPLE^*(\mathcal{L}, k, \alpha, \mathbf{u})$ when pre-computed segmentation weights $\mathbf{u}$ are used for initialization.

3   Experiments

Data and Validation. We evaluate the proposed framework and compare
fusion methods using a set of 120 atlases with manual expert reference annotations. They cover four modalities (30 T1-weighted magnetic resonance (MRT1)
images, 30 T1-weighted contrast enhanced fat saturated magnetic resonance
images (MRT1cefs), 30 computed tomography scans (CT) and 30 contrast
enhanced computed tomography (CTce) scans) with up to 20 annotated structures in each volume[1] MRT1 volumes have a field–of–view of the whole human
body (voxels: $1.1 - 1.3 \times 1.1 - 1.3 \times 6 - 7$ mm), MRT1cefs volumes of the
abdomen $(1.2 - 1.3 \times 1.2 - 1.3 \times 3$ mm), CT scans of the whole human body
$(0.8 - 0.9 \times 0.8 - 0.9 \times 1.5$ mm) and CTce scans include the chest and the abdomen
$(0.6 - 0.7 \times 0.6 - 0.7 \times 1.2 - 1.5$ mm).

Algorithmic segmentations are available from participants of the *VISCERAL
Anatomy* 2 & 3 challenges[2], where 9 groups contributed algorithms for structures
in CT and CTce and 2 in MRT1 and MRT1cefs volumes [6,11]. Each participant has been able to submit up to 5 different parameter configurations, resulting in 20 independent algorithmic estimates in CT and CTce and 2 in MRT1
and MRT1cefs volumes. Most algorithms incorporate atlas based segmentation
approaches [5,9,10,12,13], but are also based on shape and appearance modelling [7,20,25], anatomy based reasoning [4,23] or use graph cuts and spatial
relations [14]. All methods are trained on 20 atlases of each modality which are
excluded from the test set [6,11].

Since only $\mathcal{P}$ are independent for each target volume, but a sub-set of atlases
has to be used for generating $\mathcal{A}$ and for estimating the performance of each
algorithmic annotator, we performed leave-one-out cross validation on 10 atlases
of each modality resulting in a test set of 40 volumes. Each atlas of the test set
was selected once as target image and held out of the source atlas set and from
the performance estimation process. Accuracy for all structures is reported as
the Dice between segmentation estimate and gold corpus annotation [3].

Registration. Annotations are propagated from atlases to target images based
on NMI driven multiresolution affine- and non-rigid registration. We use the
NiftyReg toolbox[3], with a CUDA based implementation for affine alignment
and B-spline based non-rigid registration. For CTce volumes a spline grid with
7 mm, for CT with 9 mm, for MRT1cefs with 9 mm and for MRT1 a grid with
7 mm spacing is applied.

---

[1] Structures and RadlexIDs: r./l. lungs - RID 1302/1326, liver 58, r./l. kidneys
29662/29663, gallbladder 187, trachea 1247, aorta 480, first lumbar vertebra 29193,
r./l. adrenal gland 30324/30325, r./l. psoas major 32248/32249, muscle body of r./l.
rectus abdominis 40357/40358, pancreas 170, spleen 86, sternum 2473, urinary bladder 237 and thyroid gland 7578. For Radlex terminology refer to http://www.radlex.
org/.

[2] Organized by the EU FP7 funded project VISCERAL: http://www.visceral.eu.

[3] http://www.nitrc.org/projects/niftyreg/.

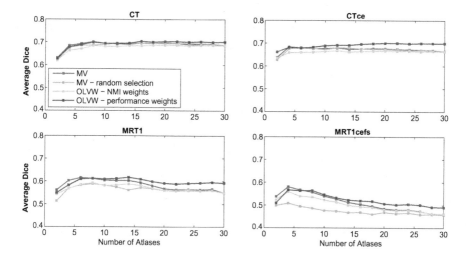

Fig. 2. Segmentation performances of *MV, MV - random selection, OLVW - NMI weights* and *OLVW - performance weights* averaged over all structures of each modalitiy evaluated for different numbers (x-axis) of selected atlases. *OLVW - performance weights* yields best results in all four modalities. (Color figure online)

Fusion Approaches. Method identifiers (*MV, OLWV, STAPLE, SIMPLE*) and input parameters follow those in Sect. 2. Depending on the input data, the method identifier is appended by letter A (atlases) if $\mathcal{L} = \mathcal{A}$, by P (participating algorithms) if $\mathcal{L} = \mathcal{P}$ and AP if $\mathcal{L} = \langle \mathcal{A}, \mathcal{P} \rangle$ (atlases and algorithms). Corresponding weights are calculated following Sect. 2.3. For SIMPLE, the number of iterations in which no segmentation is discarded is $k = 3$, similar to [18] and we set $\alpha = 1.25$ [17].

4   Results

Atlas Selection and Weighting. First, we evaluate the effect of different numbers of weighted atlases without using algorithmic segmentations. Figure 2 compares majority voting of pre-registration selected atlases (*MV*), majority voting of randomly selected atlases (*MV - random selection*), OLVW with weights derived by NMI of the transformed atlas image and the target image (*OLVW - NMI weights*) and OLVW with performance weights calculated according to Sect. 2.3 (*OLVW - performance weights*). We show the Dice coefficients averaged over all structures for each modality and increasing numbers of atlases. While all methods yield comparable results on CT volumes, differences become visible in CTce and especially in MRT1 and MRT1cefs volumes. Results show that *MV* slightly outperforms *MV - random selection* as well as *OLWV - NMI weights*. Best results in all modalities are obtained by a weighted vote that incorporates performances weights (*OLWV - performance weights*). Results furthermore show

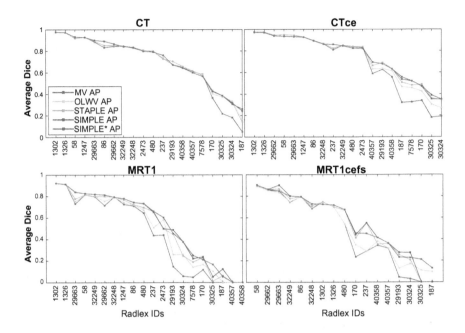

Fig. 3. Average segmentation performances of different fusion approaches that incorporate propagated atlases and algorithmic segmentation estimates on all modalities evaluated. *SIMPLE* segmentation yields in the best overall segmentation performances. Injecting reliability estimates (*SIMPLE**) results in similar performances compared to *SIMPLE* without initial segmentation weights. (Color figure online)

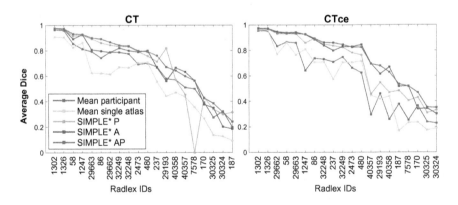

Fig. 4. Average accuracies of single algorithmic segmentations, atlases and different fusion approaches. Fusing segmentation estimates of both, atlases and algorithms (*SIMPLE* AP*) outperforms segmentations obtained by fusing estimates of one of both components (*SIMPLE* A*, *SIMPLE* P*). (Color figure online)

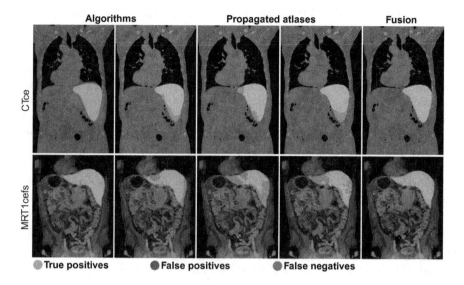

Fig. 5. Consensus plots of two algorithmic segmentation estimates, two mapped atlases and the resulting fusion of two liver segmentations obtained by *SIMPLE* AP*. (Color figure online)

an initial performance increase with an increasing amount of considered atlases followed by a constant (CT, CTce) or even decreasing segmentation performance when considering many poor atlases (MRT1, MRT1cefs).

Comparing Label Fusion Methods Integrating Atlases and Algorithms.
Figure 3 compares different label fusion approaches (*MV, OLWV, STAPLE* and *SIMPLE*) and the impact of performance based weights on the SIMPLE approach (indicated by * in the legend) on test set segmentation accuracy. Here, all methods take atlases and segmentations of participants into account. Based on the results shown in Fig. 2, we select the top 16 ranked atlases for CT, 20 for CTce, 14 for MRT1 and 8 for MRT1cefs volumes. The y-axis depicts average Dice [3] coefficients, the x-axis identifies anatomical structures, ordered by accuracy of the best performing approach.

All methods perform comparably for structures with high overall segmentation accuracy (e.g., the lungs in CT, CTce and MRT1). The benefit of weighting becomes visible for structures with lower overall segmentation accuracy, and is highest in MRT1 and MRT1cefs. Here, *OLWV AP* outperforms *MV AP* in the majority of tested structures. That is, taking the split of annotators into experts and algorithms into account does improve accuracy. Fusing segmentations with *STAPLE AP* and *SIMPLE AP* improves segmentation accuracy for all investigated structures. Excluding poorly performing segmentations (*SIMPLE AP*) results in higher segmentation accuracy, again especially in structures with low overall segmentation quality. Using reliability estimates of each contributing segmentation to initialize SIMPLE (*SIMPLE* AP*) and SIMPLE without applying initial weights (*SIMPLE AP*) reach similar segmentation performances, which is plausible since SIMPLE is reported to be independent to initial segmentation weights [18]. Small performance gains are observed in some structures of MRT1 and MRT1cefs volumes.

Multiple Atlases vs. Multiple Algorithms. Figure 4 compares average segmentation accuracies of individual atlases or individual algorithms with segmentations obtained by fusing atlases (*SIMPLE* A*), algorithms (*SIMPLE* P*) or both (*SIMPLE* AP*). As expected, all fusion approaches consistently outperform individual segmentations. Using atlases and algorithms jointly improves segmentation accuracies in the majority of structures compared to fusing algorithms or atlases only. Figure 5 illustrates the effect of fusing atlases and algorithms on liver segmentations. True positive, false negative and false positive segmented voxels of two algorithms, two propagated atlases and the resulting fused segmentation are shown in a CTce and a MRT1cefs volume.

The Resulting Silver Corpus. Finally we apply the best performing fusion method *SIMPLE* AP* to 264 additional volumes of the modalities (62 CT, 65

Table 1. Segmentation performances (μ, σ) obtained by *SIMPLE* AP*, evaluated on 10 annotated test set volumes (i.e. which were not included in algorithm training) per modality and number of silver corpus annotations (#) computed on additional volumes that will be available as a resource for the research community at www.visceral.eu.

Radlex ID	Name	CT			CTce			MRT1			MRT1cefs		
		#	μ	σ	#	μ	σ	#	μ	σ	#	μ	σ
58	liver	59	0.93	0.01	63	0.94	0.01	66	0.83	0.07	71	0.90	0.03
86	spleen	55	0.89	0.06	63	0.89	0.07	65	0.74	0.11	71	0.79	0.18
170	pancreas	57	0.43	0.19	60	0.47	0.18	63	0.21	0.21	71	0.46	0.13
187	gallbladder	40	0.24	0.19	49	0.54	0.15	46	0.05	0.05	61	0.13	0.20
237	urinary bladder	58	0.76	0.15	64	0.86	0.06	59	0.66	0.28	70	0.45	0.25
480	aorta	58	0.79	0.04	63	0.82	0.05	65	0.73	0.07	71	0.68	0.02
1247	trachea	57	0.93	0.02	62	0.93	0.02	63	0.78	0.10	-	-	-
1302	r. lung	60	0.98	0.01	64	0.97	0.01	66	0.92	0.02	-	-	-
1326	l. lung	61	0.97	0.01	63	0.97	0.01	66	0.91	0.03	-	-	-
2473	sternum	55	0.80	0.04	63	0.83	0.07	64	0.60	0.00	-	-	-
7578	thyroid gland	57	0.57	0.10	62	0.52	0.13	64	0.25	0.15	-	-	-
29193	first lumbar vertebra	57	0.67	0.36	63	0.68	0.34	58	0.46	0.25	71	0.23	0.12
29662	r. kidneys	57	0.87	0.12	63	0.94	0.01	65	0.81	0.11	71	0.86	0.18
29663	l. kidneys	58	0.90	0.03	63	0.93	0.02	64	0.84	0.06	71	0.85	0.20
30324	r. adrenal gland	54	0.32	0.20	56	0.35	0.14	50	0.38	0.14	60	0.23	0.11
30325	l. adrenal gland	54	0.36	0.19	53	0.35	0.17	41	0.17	0.22	49	0.21	0.12
32248	r. psoas major	58	0.84	0.02	63	0.86	0.02	65	0.79	0.06	71	0.73	0.12
32249	l. psoas major	56	0.84	0.02	63	0.85	0.05	65	0.82	0.06	71	0.80	0.05
40357	r. rectus abdominis	56	0.60	0.21	63	0.69	0.16	-	-	-	-	-	-
40358	l. rectus abdominis	55	0.64	0.14	64	0.63	0.17	-	-	-	-	-	-
Σ		**1122**			**1227**			**1095**			**879**		

CTce, 66 MRT1, 71 MRT1cefs) for which segmentation estimates could be generated using the algorithms submitted to *VISCERAL Anatomy* 2 & 3, resulting in the **VISCERAL Anatomy Silver Corpus** that consists a set of 4323 segmentations of anatomical structures which will be available as a resource for the research community at www.visceral.eu.

For reference, Table 1 lists the number of computed segmentations (#) of all target structures in each modality as well as average segmentation performances (μ) and corresponding standard deviations (σ) which serve as structure and modality specific segmentation performance estimates of generated silver corpus annotations.

5 Conclusion

Algorithmic segmentation of anatomical structures is essential for computer aided diagnosis, since large scale manual annotation is infeasible. Benchmarks that evaluate multiple algorithms on medical imaging data contribute critically to assessing their accuracy, and thereby advancing method research. At the same time the variety and number of these algorithms can be leveraged to create large scale *silver corpora* of imaging data annotated by some sort of consensus of these contributions. Here, we propose and evaluate a framework for creating silver corpus annotations of large scale data. We first apply a number of different segmentation algorithms that were entries to an anatomy segmentation challenge to segment the data. Then, we fuse labels transferred from manually annotated atlases and the labels obtained by the algorithmic segmentations. The results demonstrate that adding algorithmic estimators improves accuracy compared to baseline segmentations obtained by mere expert atlas fusion. Furthermore, informing the label fusion by weighting algorithmic and atlas segmentations based on their accuracy in comparison to expert annotations improves accuracy over standard label fusion techniques. The accuracy gained by fusion is highest for anatomical structures on which algorithms perform poorly. Analogously, even though fusion of algorithmic segmentations is already beneficial across the entire range of organs, adding atlases furthermore improves accuracy for structures where algorithms have low accuracy. We applied the best performing method, *SIMPLE* AP* (fusing atlases and algorithmic segmentations, initialized with performance estimate weights), to a dataset of 264 volumes of four modalities (CT, CTce, MRT1, MRT1cefs). This resulted in a set of 4323 silver corpus annotations, which will be available for the research community at www.visceral.eu.

Acknowledgements. The research leading to these results has received funding from the European Union Seventh Framework Programme (FP7/2007-2013) under grant agreements 318068 (VISCERAL) and 257528 (KHRESMOI). We furthermore acknowledge the support of NVIDIA Corporation with the donation of a Tesla K40 GPU used for this work and would like to thank all research groups contributing to this work by participating in the *VISCERAL Anatomy* 2 & 3 benchmarks [4,5,7,9,10,12–14,20,23,25].

References

1. Aljabar, P., Heckemann, R.A., Hammers, A., Hajnal, J.V., Rueckert, D.: Multi-atlas based segmentation of brain images: atlas selection and its effect on accuracy. NeuroImage **46**(3), 726–738 (2009)
2. Artaechevarria, X., Munoz-Barrutia, A., Ortiz-de Solórzano, C.: Combination strategies in multi-atlas image segmentation: application to brain mr data. IEEE Trans. Med. Imaging **28**(8), 1266–1277 (2009)
3. Dice, L.R.: Measures of the amount of ecologic association between species. Ecology **26**(3), 297–302 (1945)
4. Dicente Cid, Y., Depeursinge, A., Jiménez del Toro, O.A., Müller, H.: Efficient and fully automatic segmentation of the lungs in ct volumes. In: Goksel, O., Jiménez-del Toro, O.A., Foncubierta-Rodríguez, A., Müller, H. (eds.) Proceedings of the VISCERAL Challenge at ISBI, vol. 1390, p. 31, April 2015
5. Gass, T., Szekely, G., Goksel, O.: Multi-atlas segmentation and landmark localization in images with large field of view. In: Menze, B., Langs, G., Montillo, A., Kelm, M., Müller, H., Zhang, S., Cai, W.T., Metaxas, D. (eds.) MCV 2014. LNCS, vol. 8848, pp. 171–180. Springer, Heidelberg (2014)
6. Göksel, O., Jiménez-del Toro, O.A., Foncubierta-Rodríguez, A., Muller, H.: Overview of the VISCERAL challenge at ISBI 2015. In: Göksel, O., Jiménez-del Toro, O.A., Foncubierta-Rodríguez, A., Müller, H. (eds.) Proceedings of the VISCERAL Challenge at ISBI, New York, NY, May 2015
7. He, B., Huang, C., Jia, F.: Fully automatic multi-organ segmentation based on multi-boost learning and statistical shape model search. In: Goksel, O., Jiménez-del Toro, O.A., Foncubierta-Rodríguez, A., Müller, H. (eds.) Proceedings of the VISCERAL Challenge at ISBI, vol. 1390, pp. 18–21, April 2015
8. Heckemann, R.A., Hajnal, J.V., Aljabar, P., Rueckert, D., Hammers, A.: Automatic anatomical brain MRI segmentation combining label propagation and decision fusion. NeuroImage **33**(1), 115–126 (2006)
9. Heinrich, M.P., Maier, O., Handels, H.: Multi-modal multi-atlas segmentation using discrete optimisation and self-similarities. In: Goksel, O., Jiménez-del Toro, O.A., Foncubierta-Rodríguez, A., Müller, H. (eds.) Proceedings of the VISCERAL Challenge at ISBI, vol. 1390, p. 27, April 2015
10. Jiménez del Toro, O.A., Dicente Cid, Y., Depeursinge, A., Müller, H., Hierarchic anatomical structure segmentation guided by spatial correlations (anatseg-gspac): Visceral anatomy3. In: Goksel, O., Jiménez-del Toro, O.A., Foncubierta-Rodríguez, A., Müller, H. (eds.) Proceedings of the VISCERAL Challenge at ISBI, vol. 1390, pp. 22–66. CEUR-WS, April 2015. http://ceur-ws.org
11. Jiménez del Toro, O.A., Goksel, O., Menze, B., Müller, H., Langs, G., Weber, M.A., Eggel, I., Gruenberg, K., Holzer, M., Jakab, A., Kotsios-Kontokotsios, G., Krenn, M., Salas Fernandez, T., Schaer, R., Abdel Aziz, T., Winterstein, M., Hanbury, A.: Visceral-visual concept extraction challenge in radiology: ISBI 2014 challenge organization. In: Göksel, O. (ed.) Proceedings of the VISCERAL Challenge at ISBI. CEUR Workshop Proceedings, pp. 6–15 (2014)
12. Jiménez del Toro, O.A., Müller, H.: Hierarchic Multi-atlas based segmentation for anatomical structures: evaluation in the VISCERAL anatomy benchmarks. In: Menze, B., Langs, G., Montillo, A., Kelm, M., Müller, H., Zhang, S., Cai, W.T., Metaxas, D. (eds.) MCV 2014. LNCS, vol. 8848, pp. 189–200. Springer, Heidelberg (2014)

13. Kahl, F., Alvén, J., Enqvist, O., Fejne, F., Ulén, J., Fredriksson, J., Landgren, M., Larsson, V.: Good features for reliable registration in multi-atlas segmentation. In: Goksel, O., Jiménez-del Toro, O.A., Foncubierta-Rodríguez, A., Müller, H. (eds.) Proceedings of the VISCERAL Challenge at ISBI, vol. 1390, pp. 12–17, April 2015

14. Kéchichian, R., Valette, S., Sdika, M., Desvignes, M.: Automatic 3D multiorgan segmentation via clustering and graph cut using spatial relations and hierarchically-registered atlases. In: Menze, B., Langs, G., Montillo, A., Kelm, M., Müller, H., Zhang, S., Cai, W.T., Metaxas, D. (eds.) MCV 2014. LNCS, vol. 8848, pp. 201–209. Springer, Heidelberg (2014)

15. Kittler, J., Alkoot, F.M.: Sum versus vote fusion in multiple classifier systems. IEEE Trans. Pattern Anal. Mach. Intell. 25(1), 110–115 (2003)

16. Kittler, J., Hatef, M., Duin, R.P.W., Matas, J.: On combining classifiers. IEEE Trans. Pattern Anal. Mach. Intell. 20(3), 226–239 (1998)

17. Klein, S., Staring, M., Murphy, K., Viergever, M., Pluim, J.P.W.: Elastix: a toolbox for intensity-based medical image registration. IEEE Trans. Med. Imaging 29(1), 196–205 (2010)

18. Langerak, T.R., Van der Heide, U.A., Kotte, A.N.T.J., Viergever, M.A., Van Vulpen, M., Pluim, J.P.W.: Label fusion in atlas-based segmentation using a selective and iterative method for performance level estimation (simple). IEEE Trans. Med. Imaging 29(12), 2000–2008 (2010)

19. Langs, G., Hanbury, A., Menze, B., Müller, H.: VISCERAL: towards large data in medical imaging — challenges and directions. In: Greenspan, H., Müller, H., Syeda-Mahmood, T. (eds.) MCBR-CDS 2012. LNCS, vol. 7723, pp. 92–98. Springer, Heidelberg (2013)

20. Li, X., Huang, C., Jia, F., Li, Z., Fang, C., Fan, Y.: Automatic liver segmentation using statistical prior models and free-form deformation. In: Menze, B., Langs, G., Montillo, A., Kelm, M., Müller, H., Zhang, S., Cai, W.T., Metaxas, D. (eds.) MCV 2014. LNCS, vol. 8848, pp. 181–188. Springer, Heidelberg (2014)

21. Rohlfing, T., Brandt, R., Menzel, R., Maurer, C.R.: Evaluation of atlas selection strategies for atlas-based image segmentation with application to confocal microscopy images of bee brains. NeuroImage 21(4), 1428–1442 (2004)

22. Roli, F., Kittler, J., Fumera, G., Muntoni, D.: An experimental comparison of classifier fusion rules for multimodal personal identity verification systems. In: Roli, F., Kittler, J. (eds.) MCS 2002. LNCS, vol. 2364, pp. 325–335. Springer, Heidelberg (2002)

23. Spanier, A.B., Joskowicz, L.: Rule-based ventral cavity multi-organ automatic segmentation in CT scans. In: Menze, B., Langs, G., Montillo, A., Kelm, M., Müller, H., Zhang, S., Cai, W.T., Metaxas, D. (eds.) MCV 2014. LNCS, vol. 8848, pp. 163–170. Springer, Heidelberg (2014)

24. Studholme, C., Hill, D.L.G., Hawkes, D.J.: An overlap invariant entropy measure of 3D medical image alignment. Pattern recognition 32(1), 71–86 (1999)

25. Wang, C., Smedby, O.: Automatic multi-organ segmentation using fast model based level set method and hierarchical shape priors. In: Goksel, O., Jiménez-del Toro, O.A., Foncubierta-Rodríguez, A., Müller, H. (eds.) Proceedings of the VISCERAL Challenge at ISBI, vol. 1194, pp. 25–31 (2014)

26. Warfield, S.K., Zou, K.H., Wells III, W.M.: Validation of image segmentation and expert quality with an expectation-maximization algorithm. In: Dohi, T., Kikinis, R. (eds.) MICCAI 2002, Part I. LNCS, vol. 2488, pp. 298–306. Springer, Heidelberg (2002)

Psoas Major Muscle Segmentation Using Higher-Order Shape Prior

Tsutomu Inoue[1(✉)], Yoshiro Kitamura[1,2], Yuanzhong Li[1],
Wataru Ito[1], and Hiroshi Ishikawa[2,3]

[1] Imaging Technology Center, Fujifilm Corporation, Tokyo, Japan
`tsutomu.inoue@fujifilm.com`
[2] Department of Computer Science and Engineering,
Waseda University, Tokyo, Japan
[3] JST CREST, Tokyo, Japan

Abstract. We propose a novel segmentation method based on higher-order graph cuts which enables the utilization of prior knowledge regarding anatomical shapes. We applied the method for segmentation of psoas major muscles by using combinations of logistic curves which representing their shapes. The higher-order terms consisting of variables (voxels) just inside or outside of the estimated shapes are added to the energy function to encourage the segmentation results to fit to the shapes. We verified the effectiveness of the method with 20 abdominal CT images. By comparing the segmentation results to the ground truth data prepared by a clinical expert, we validated the method where it achieved the Jaccard similarity coefficient (JSC) of 75.4 % (right major) and 77.5 % (left major). We also confirmed that the proposed method worked well for thick CT images.

Keywords: Psoas major muscle · Abdominal CT images · Graph cuts · Higher-order potential

1 Introduction

Muscle mass of the body is known as an important predictive factor of health and prognostic of surgery [1]. For instance, the survival rate of surgeries decreases as a patient loses muscle mass [2]. Although people may try to keep muscle mass as much as they can, someone may suffer from sarcopenia, i.e., the loss of muscles as a result of aging. Muscles are categorized into inner and outer groups. The former functions to move the body, while the latter mainly keeps the body balance. In the clinical practice, the psoas major muscle, which is one of the inner muscles, is used as an indicator of the muscle mass of the whole body. However, the accuracy of the measurement is currently not reliable enough because the muscle mass is measured in a 2D axial CT image, which can be chosen differently in each hospital. Although measuring the whole muscle in 3D could improve the accuracy, it has not become common since 3D measurement, especially segmentation, is a time consuming task.

Figure 1 shows the entirety of psoas major. It originates from the last thoracic vertebra (T12) along with the five lumbar vertebrae (L1–L5) and reaches the lesser

© Springer International Publishing Switzerland 2016
B. Menze et al. (Eds.): MCV Workshop 2015, LNCS 9601, pp. 116–124, 2016.
DOI: 10.1007/978-3-319-42016-5_11

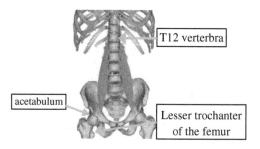

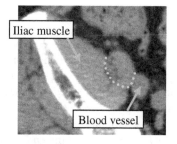

Fig. 1. The psoas major muscle and bone in the 3D image. It is originated from the side of T12 and its end is located in the lesser trochanter of the femur.

Fig. 2. The psoas major muscle seen in an axial slice. The dotted lines indicate the psoas major region: the red shows apparent edge, and the yellow obscure edge. (Color figure online)

trochanter of the femur. There is a pair of the muscles on both sides of the body. Automatic segmentation of the psoas major is difficult, because they are in contact with surrounding organs which appear with almost the same intensities: Fig. 2 shows an example of an axial image of the psoas major that is surrounded by the iliac muscle and blood vessels.

A few methods have been presented to tackle the problem. In [3], the psoas major muscle is segmented using a 3D shape model with an approximated function learned from test cases. They estimated the spindle-like structure between the last thoracic vertebra (T12) and the lacuna musculorum insertion by a quadratic function with two parameters. On the other hand, Meesters [4] presented a multi-atlas-based segmentation with a weighted decision fusion and the non-rigid registration.

In this paper, we present a novel segmentation method based on graph cuts. The method can utilize prior knowledge regarding anatomical shapes by using higher order potentials. A segmentation method utilizing higher-order shape prior has been applied for extracting blood vessels [5]. In contrast to [5], which modeled circular shapes, our method models the spindle-like shape of the psoas major that varies depending on the patient. The spindle-like shape is parameterized through logistics curves. We prepare multiple candidate shapes to deal with the wide variety of shapes depending on the patient. Each candidate shape is encoded in a submodular higher-order potential to encourage a set of voxels to entirely fall inside or outside of each candidate by having the same label. The multiple candidates are added into the graph-cut framework. The higher-order potential has the effect of lowering the energy if and only if all of the voxel variables belonging to the potential have the same label. Thus only candidates that match to the segmentation results contribute to lowering the energy. We show the effectiveness of the proposed method by a comparison with the ground truth data prepared by a radiologist.

2 Method

Our goal is a fully automatic segmentation method of the psoas major muscle in CT images. The proposed method consists of the two steps shown in Fig. 3. The first step extracts the centerline of the psoas major. The centerline is a spline curve defined by the three control points: *start*, *middle* and *end*. In this paper, we confine the muscle regions to be extracted to the range from the side of T12 to the level of the axial image where the acetabulum is seen. The upper end corresponds to the *start* point, and the lower end corresponds to the *end* point. The *middle* point is between the *start* and the *end* points. The *start* and the *end* points are detected based on the vertebrae labeling (Sect. 2.1.1). The *middle* point is determined by pre-segmentation of the psoas major region around the middle of the centerline (Sect. 2.1.2). In the second step, the stacked 3D MPR image is generated along the centerline. Then the psoas major region is segmented by using higher-order graph cuts. The psoas shape model we utilize in the graph cuts is described in Sect. 2.2. Finally, we describe how we give the energy function including the higher-order potentials in Sect. 2.3.

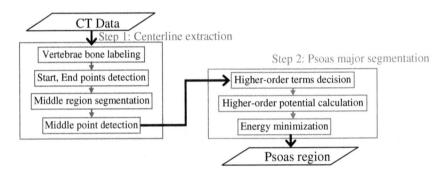

Fig. 3. Flowchart of the proposed method

2.1 Psoas Major Centerline Creation

2.1.1 Start and End Points Detection

We start by describing how to detect the *start* and the *end* points of the muscle. The *start* point is determined by vertebral bone labeling. First, the centerline of the vertebral bones is extracted by the vertebra detector based on machine learning described in [6]. Next, the T12 vertebra position is found by counting the number of vertebrae from the lowest vertebra. Next, the femur bone head is found by a detector which has learned the appearance of the circular shape of the bone head. The ilium regions are extracted by binarizing process of high CT value regions that surround the detected femur bone head (Fig. 4). Finally, the *end* point is determined as the right upper side of the ilium region.

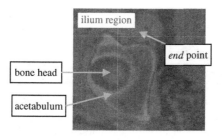

Fig. 4. The *end* point of the psoas major is detected from the segmented bone region on the slice shown in the top of the bone head.

2.1.2 Middle Point Detection

We detect the *middle* point by pre-segmentation of the psoas major regions on an oblique plane that crosses the midpoint of the centerline and orthogonal to the direction of the centerline. The region of interest (ROI) is set around the midpoint. The muscle region in the ROI is extracted using the standard first-order graph cut, which minimizes an energy function represented as

$$E(L) = \sum_{p \in P} D_p(f_p) + \sum_{(p,q) \in N} D_{p,q}(f_p, f_q), \tag{1}$$

where N is the set of neighboring pairs of voxels and f_p represents a binary label which takes 0 (background) or 1 (foreground), defined for each voxel p. The functions $D_p(f_p)$ and $D_p(f_p, f_q)$ are zeroth- and first-order potentials for the label f_p, and the label pair (f_p, f_q), respectively.

In our implementation, the zeroth-order potential is given by the following equation:

$$D_p(f_p) = \begin{cases} -\alpha & \text{if } f_p = 0 \land (I(p) < T_1 \lor I(p) > T_2 \lor d(p,c) > C_1) \\ -\alpha & \text{if } f_p = 1 \land I(p) > T_3 \land I(p) < T_4 \land d(p,c) < C_2 \\ 0 & \text{otherwise} \end{cases} \tag{2}$$

Here, $I(p)$ is the image intensity (i.e., the CT value) of voxel p, T_i are threshold values for image intensity, $d(p,c)$ is a distance between voxel p and the center c of the ROI, and C_i are threshold values for the distance. Since we can assume that the muscle region is near the center of the ROI, this function is designed to take a low value when (i) a voxel that is close to the center takes the foreground label or (ii) a voxel that is far from the center takes the background label.

The first-order potential is given by

$$D_{p,q}(f_p, f_q) = \begin{cases} f_1 \left(|I(p) - I(q)| + |\nabla^2 I(p) - \nabla^2 I(q)| \right) \cdot f_2 \left(\dfrac{I(p) + I(q)}{2} - I_{\text{average}} \right) \\ \qquad \cdot f_3 \left(\dfrac{\nabla^2 I(p) + \nabla^2 I(q)}{2} \right) \Big/ \left(\dfrac{d(p,c) + d(q,c)}{2} \right) & \text{if } f_p \neq f_q \\ 0 & \text{otherwise,} \end{cases} \tag{3}$$

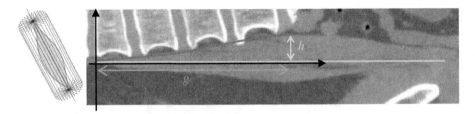

Fig. 5. (LEFT) The configuration of the psoas muscle model. (RIGHT) One of the oblique planes and the logistic curve that models the psoas muscle. In the left figure, the orange region shows the psoas muscle. The blue line shows the centerline. Each black quadrangles illustrates the oblique plane. In the right figure, the red curve shows the logistic curve that models the shape of the psoas muscle. The blue line shows the centerline of the psoas muscle. The yellow and green arrows indicate the estimated radius and half of the length of the centerline of the psoas muscle, respectively. (Color figure online)

where f_1, f_2, and f_3 are monotonically decreasing functions, $\nabla^2 I(p)$ represents the Laplasian value at voxel p, and I_{average} is an average intensity value of the voxels on the centerline. The middle point of the centerline is obtained as the center of the regions segmented by minimizing the energy function. Note that the average distance from the center to the boundaries (D_{pre}) and the average intensity value (I_{pre}) of the segmented regions are also calculated for later use in constructing the psoas major model.

2.2   Psoas Major Model

Even though the psoas major generally has a spindle-like shape, the variation in its three-dimensional shape is very wide. To reduce the computational cost, we use a decomposed 2D model. We consider multiple oblique planes passing through the centerline in the 3D image as shown on the left in Fig. 5. On each plane, the psoas major is assumed to form a semicircular shape. Each curve parameterized by i and j is represented by a logistic function of the form,

$$f_{i,j}(t) = \frac{h + \tau_i}{1 + \exp\big((0.2g \cdot (t_j - t) + t_j - 20)\big/(20 - t_j)\big)}, \tag{4}$$

where g is a half of the length of the centerline and h is the height of the logistic curve at the middle point of the centerline, which in turn is determined according to the value D_{pre} calculated in Sect. 2.1.2. To represent a wide variation of the psoas muscle shapes, a number of logistic curves is prepared by changing τ_i and t_j on each plane. Note that the oblique planes are set every 15 ° around the centerline.

2.3   Psoas Major Segmentation

The psoas major regions are segmented from the stacked MPR images along the centerline by minimizing the higher-order energy function defined by

$$E(L) = \sum_{p \in P} D_p(f_p) + \sum_{p,q \in N} D_{p,q}(f_p, f_q) + \sum_{s \in S} D_s(f_s), \qquad (5)$$

where the first and the second terms are zeroth- and first-order potentials similar to those in Eq. (1), while $D_s(f_s)$ represents a higher-order potential determined by the estimated shape of psoas major, where s is a set of voxels that form the candidate shape, S is a set of such sets, and f_s is the vector of binary values at the voxels belonging to s.

The zeroth-order term is given by the same function as in Eq. (2):

$$D_p(f_p) = \begin{cases} -\alpha & \text{if} \quad f_p = 0 \wedge (I(p) < T_1 \vee I(p) > T_2 \vee d(p,c) > C_1) \\ -\alpha & \text{if} \quad f_p = 1 \wedge I(p) > T_3 \wedge I(p) < T_4 \wedge d(p,c) < C_2 \\ 0 & \text{otherwise} \end{cases}, \qquad (6)$$

where T_1 and T_2 are the lower and upper bounds for distinguishing the muscle regions from other structures, determined by adding or subtracting a constant to the value I_{pre} from the pre-segmentation step. The thresholds C_1 and C_2 for distance are determined similarly from the estimated radius D_{pre}.

The first-order term is given by

$$D_{p,q}(f_p, f_q) = \begin{cases} f_1(|I(p) - I(q)|) \cdot f_2\left(\left|\frac{I(p)+I(q)}{2} - I_{pre}\right|\right) \Big/ \left(\frac{d(p,c)+d(q,c)}{2}\right) & \text{if } f_p \neq f_q \\ 0 & \text{otherwise} \end{cases}, \qquad (7)$$

where f_1 and f_2 are monotonically decreasing functions.

The higher order term $D_s(f_s)$ is a function of the form

$$D_s(f_s) = \min\left\{ \alpha, \quad \sum_{p \in s; f_p \neq l} \cdot \frac{\alpha}{N} \right\}. \qquad (8)$$

This function takes a low value if and only if all but at most N of the variables f_p at the voxels in the term have the target label l. It gives an increasing penalty as more variables violate the condition, until it saturates at N violating variables. This is called the robust P^n model in [7]. To set a shape prior based on this function, we choose the set of variables (voxels) s from inside or outside the candidate shape. The voxels inside the shape are encouraged to have the foreground label $l = 1$, while the voxels outside are encouraged to have the background label $l = 0$. Thus, the two types of higher order potentials are added in pairs into the energy function per candidate shape. We set multiple candidates changing the parameters τ_i and t_j in Eq. (4).

An important factor is how to set the weight α depending on the candidate shape and the given image. We define the weights α_{inside} and $\alpha_{outside}$ for the paired inside and outside terms, respectively, by

$$\alpha_{\text{inside}} = f\left(|\mu_{\text{inside}} - I_{\text{pre}}|\right)g\left(\max(\sigma_{\text{inside}}^2 - \sigma_{\text{pre}}^2, 0)\right), \tag{9}$$

$$\alpha_{\text{outside}} = f\left(|\mu_{\text{outside}} - I_{\text{pre}}|\right)g\left(\max(\sigma_{\text{outside}}^2 - \sigma_{\text{pre}}^2, \sigma_{\text{outside}}^2 - \sigma_{\text{inside}}^2, 0)\right), \tag{10}$$

where μ_{inside} and σ_{inside}^2 respectively represent the average and the variance of the intensities at the voxels belonging to the inside term, whereas μ_{outside} and $\sigma_{\text{outside}}^2$ are those for the outside term. Also, I_{pre} and σ_{pre}^2 are the average and the variance of the intensities in the pre-segmented region, respectively. The functions f and g are monotonically increasing functions. In the experiments, N is set to 10 % of the total number of voxels in s.

3   Experimental Result and Discussion

For validation, we used 20 abdominal CT images. The dataset consists of CT images of 14 males (28–93 years old) and 6 females (22–87 years old). The slice thicknesses of those are from 1.0 to 5.0 mm. The voxel sizes are from 0.625^2 to 0.976^2 mm^2. The ground truth segmentation data was prepared manually by a clinical expert.

The segmentation accuracies were evaluated by Jaccard similarity coefficient (JSC). JSC is the ratio of the volume of the intersection of the ground truth region A and the segmentation results B to that of their union,

$$JSC = \frac{|A \cap B|}{|A \cup B|}. \tag{11}$$

The summary of the evaluation results are shown in Fig. 6. Though the thicknesses of the CT images vary from case to case, it can be seen that the method performs reasonably well for the entire dataset. The processing time was 10.22 to 33.58 s per case on a quad-core 3.4 GHz PC. The average JSCs were 75.4 % for right major and 77.5 % for the left major, respectively. Figure 7 shows the case where the proposed method is successful. Almost all psoas major regions have been segmented without incorrectly including other surrounding structures. We can see that the psoas major in the red circle were separated well from the vessels. Figure 8 shows a comparison of the segmentation results obtained by the methods with and without the higher-order potentials. We can see that the method with the shape prior generated better results, since the shape term prevented including the neighboring vessels or muscles. Figure 9 shows an example of failure cases. The method segmented the kidney and vessels with smooth curves according to the shape prior. The reason is that the features such as the intensity average and variance used to determine the higher-order potentials could not distinguish the psoas major from other structures.

We could not directly compare our method with other state-of-the-art methods because there are no common datasets available. Still, let us compare our quantitative results with those from other studies [3, 4] that evaluate the performance with the JSC of the segmented volume. It is reported that the method [3] achieved 72.3 % on

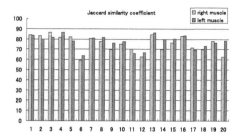

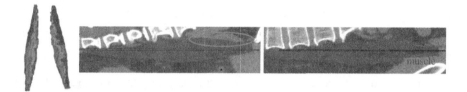

Fig. 6. The JSCs of the segmentation results of 20 test cases.

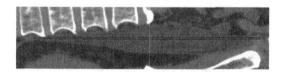

Fig. 7. Successful segmentation results of the proposed method shown in 3D and on an oblique plane. Correctly segmented regions are shown in purple, whereas missed regions and regions incorrectly segmented as muscle are shown in blue and red, respectively. (Color figure online)

Fig. 8. A comparison of the segmentation results with and without the shape prior. The yellow region was segmented as the muscle in both cases. The red region was segmented as muscle only by the method with the shape prior. The green regions were segmented as muscle only by the method without the shape prior. (Color figure online)

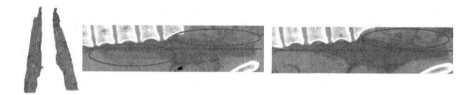

Fig. 9. Unsuccessful segmentation results of the proposed method shown in 3D and on an oblique plane. Correctly segmented regions are shown in purple, whereas regions incorrectly segmented as muscle are shown in red. (Color figure online)

80 cases, whereas [4] achieved 63.4 % (left side) and 68.6 % (right side) on 20 CT datasets. Therefore, we consider our method is competitive against these methods, as it achieves 75.4 % (left side) and 77.5 % (right side).

4 Conclusions

We proposed a novel segmentation method for psoas major muscle from CT images. The method enables the utilization of prior knowledge regarding anatomical shapes in higher-order graph cuts. The higher-order terms consisting of variables (voxels) just inside or outside of the estimated shapes are added to the energy function to encourage the segmentation results to fit to the shapes. A quantitative experimental evaluation in 20 CT cases suggests that the method is competitive against the state-of-the-art. The proposed method can segment the psoas major region as smoother shape. In the future work, we would like to decrease the misclassification of surrounding vessels and other muscles.

References

1. Martin, L., Birdsell, L., Macdonald, N., Reiman, T., Clandinin, M.T., McCargar, L.J., Murphy, R., Ghosh, S., Sawyer, M.B., Baracos, V.E.: Cancer cachexia in the age of obesty: skeletal muscle depletion is a powerful prognostic factor, independent of body mass index. J. Clin. Oncol. **31**(12), 1539–1547 (2013)
2. Wannamethee, S.G., Shaper, A.G., Whincup, P.H., Lennon, L., Papacosta, O., Sattar, N.: The obesity paradox in men with coronary heart disease and heart failure: the role of muscle mass and leptin. Int. J. Cardiol. **171**(1), 49–55 (2014)
3. Kamiya, N., Zhou, X., Chen, H., Muramatsu, C., Hara, T., Yokoyama, R., Kanematsu, M., Hoshi, H., Fujita, H.: Automated Segmentation of psoas major muscle in X-ray CT images by use of a shape model: preliminary study. Radiol. Phys. Technol. **5**(1), 5–14 (2012)
4. Meesters, S.P.L., Yokota, F., Okada, T., Takaya, M., Tomiyama, N., Yao, J., Liguraru, M.G., Summers, R.M., Sato, Y.: Multi atlas-based muscle segmentation in abdominal CT images with varying field of view. Paper presented at the International Forum on Medical Imaging in Asia (IFMIA), 16–17 November 2012
5. Kitamura, Y., Li, Y., Ito, W., Ishikawa, H.: Coronary lumen and plaque segmentation from CTA using higher-order shape prior. In: Golland, P., Hata, N., Barillot, C., Hornegger, J., Howe, R. (eds.) MICCAI 2014, Part I. LNCS, vol. 8673, pp. 339–347. Springer, Heidelberg (2014)
6. Wang, C., Li, Y., Ito, W., Shimura, K., Abe, K.: A machine learning approach to extract spinal column centerline from three-dimensional CT data. In: Proceedings of SPIE, vol. 7259, p. 72594T (2009)
7. Kohli, P., Ladicky, L., Torr, P.H.S.: Robust higher order potentials for enforcing label consistency. In: Proceedings of CVPR (2008)
8. Kadoury, S., Abi-Jaoudeh, N., Valdes, P.A.: Higher-order CRF tumor segmentation with discriminant manifold potentials. In: Mori, K., Sakuma, I., Sato, Y., Barillot, C., Navab, N. (eds.) MICCAI 2013, Part I. LNCS, vol. 8149, pp. 719–726. Springer, Heidelberg (2013)

Poster Session

Joint Feature-Sample Selection and Robust Classification for Parkinson's Disease Diagnosis

Ehsan Adeli-Mosabbeb[1], Chong-Yaw Wee[1,2], Le An[1], Feng Shi[1], and Dinggang Shen[1(✉)]

[1] Department of Radiology and BRIC, University of North Carolina at Chapel Hill, Chapel Hill, NC 27599, USA
dgshen@med.unc.edu

[2] Department of Biomedical Engineering, National University of Singapore, Singapore, Singapore

Abstract. Parkinson's disease (PD) is an overwhelming neurodegenerative disorder caused by deterioration of a neurotransmitter, known as dopamine. Lack of this chemical messenger in the brain impairs several brain regions and yields to various movement and non-motor symptoms. The incidence of PD is considered to be doubled in the next two decades and this urges more researches on its early diagnosis and treatment. In this paper, we propose an approach to diagnose PD using magnetic resonance imaging (MRI) data. We first introduce a joint feature-sample selection method to select the optimal subset of samples and features for a reliable training process. This procedure selects the most discriminative features and discards poor sample (outliers). Then, a robust classification framework is proposed that can simultaneously de-noise the selected subset of features and samples, and learn a classification model. Our model can further de-noise the test samples based on the cleaned training data. Experimental results on both synthetic and a publicly available PD dataset show promising results.

1 Introduction

Parkinson's disease (PD) is a neurodegenerative brain disorder characterized by the progressive impairment and deterioration of brain neurons. PD is caused when the brain gradually stops producing a vital endogenous chemical messenger known as dopamine. Dopamine is produced by the neurons that are concentrated in an area of brain recognized as substantia nigra. It is a neurotransmitter regulating the communication between the substantia nigra and the corpus striatum. This communication coordinates the balanced regular muscle movements. Lack of dopamine yields loss of ability to control body movements, along with some non-motor problems (*e.g.*, depression, anxiety, apathy/abulia, *etc.*) [1]. People with PD may lose up to 80 % of dopamine before symptoms appear [2,3]. Thus, early diagnosis and treatment are crucial to slow down the progression of PD in the initial stages.

Although there is no specific test for PD diagnosis, the diagnosis process includes analyzing a sequence of symptoms while eliminating other probable

© Springer International Publishing Switzerland 2016
B. Menze et al. (Eds.): MCV Workshop 2015, LNCS 9601, pp. 127–136, 2016.
DOI: 10.1007/978-3-319-42016-5_12

syndromes or causes of each single symptom. In practice, different imaging modalities could be incorporated. SPECT imaging is usually considered for the differential diagnosis of PD and often used for people with tremor [3,4]. Recently, many researches exploit MRI to analyze the changes in different regions of the brain in PD patients [1,3]. After the production of dopamine is impaired, other parts of the brain, including cortical surfaces, are also affected, thus causing the movement and non-motor symptoms [2]. Literature studies show that these influences should be characterized by specific types of MRI data [3]. In this research, we investigate the diagnosis of PD from such effects on the brain by analyzing MR images, using machine learning techniques.

MR images can be noisy due to different factors, *e.g.*, patient movements or device limitations. Most existing works manually discard poor samples by checking the images one by one. This eventually induces undesirable bias to the learned model. Therefore, it is of great interest if we could automatically select the more reliable samples, boosting up the robustness of the method and its application in a clinical setting. On the other hand, for the purposes of diagnosis, we analyze the MR images by parcellating them into several pre-defined regions of interest (ROIs) and extracting features from each ROI. The disease might not be directly associated to all of the pre-defined regions in the brain [2]. Therefore, we also need to select the most important and relevant regions for our diagnosis procedure, like in [5–7].

Unlike many previous works, in which either feature selection [6,7] or sample selection [8] is performed, or both are considered but in sequel [5], we perform a joint feature-sample selection. The two processes (or two sub-problems) affect one another, and performing one before the other does not guarantee the selection of the best overall subset of both features and samples. Thus, these two sub-problems are overlapping, but do not have optimal sub-structures [9]. In other words, optimal overall solution is not composed of optimal solution to each sub-problem. This motivates us to jointly search for the best subsets of features and samples and introduce a novel joint feature-sample selection (JFSS) method based on how well the training labels could be represented sparsely by different number of features and samples. After feature-sample selection, we further introduce a robust classification scheme, following the least-squares linear discriminant analysis (LS-LDA) [10] formulation and the robust regression scheme [11], specially designed to enhance robustness to noise. This is because MRI is prone to noise, due to many different factors in the imaging and processing stages.

2   Overview of the Proposed Method

The whole procedure is illustrated in Fig. 1. After preprocessing the subjects' MRI scans, we extract features from their pre-defined brain ROIs, and select the best subsets of features and samples through our proposed JFSS. The joint feature-sample selection procedure is able to simultaneously discard poor samples and redundant features. Here, outlier samples and samples with non-reliable predictive power for the classification purpose are considered as poor. After JFSS,

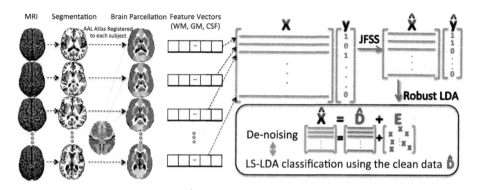

MRI   Segmentation   Brain Parcellation   Feature Vectors (WM, GM, CSF)

Fig. 1. Overview of our proposed method: First, the MR images are processed and tissue segmented images are obtained. Then, the anatomical automatic labeling (AAL) atlas is non-linearly registered to each subject's original space and the WM, GM and CSF volumes of each ROI are calculated as features. These features form $\mathbf{X}$, and the corresponding labels form $\mathbf{y}$. Through our proposed joint feature-sample selection (JFSS), we discard some uninformative features and samples, leading to $\hat{\mathbf{X}}$ and $\hat{\mathbf{y}}$. Then, we train a robust classifier (i.e., Robust LDA) in which we jointly decompose $\hat{\mathbf{X}}$ into cleaned data $\hat{\mathbf{D}}$ and its noise component $\mathbf{E}$, and classify the cleaned data.

there may still exist some noise in the remaining data. This noise is usually reflected in the feature values, which are associated with the single ROIs and not the whole sample. To further clean the data, we decompose the data to a cleaned version and its noise component. This is done in conjugation with the classification process, in a supervised manner, to increase its robustness to noise. Importantly, the test data is also de-noised by representing it as a locally compact linear combination of the cleaned training data.

The key methodological contributions in our work are three-fold: (1) We propose a new joint feature-sample selection (JFSS) procedure, which jointly selects the best subset of most discriminative features and best samples to build a classification model, based on them. (2) We utilize the robust regression method [11] to develop a robust classification model and then proposed to de-noise the test data based on supervised cleaned training samples. (3) We applied our method for PD diagnosis, as PD-data driven methods are scarce, and achieved good results.

3   Data Acquisition, Processing and Notations

The data used in this paper were obtained from the Parkinson's progression markers initiative (PPMI) database[1] [12]. PPMI is the first substantial study for identifying the PD progression biomarkers to advance the understanding of the disease. In this research, we use the MRI data acquired by the PPMI study, in which a T1-weighted, 3D sequence (e.g., MPRAGE or SPGR) is acquired

---

[1] http://www.ppmi-info.org/data.

for each subject using 3T SIEMENS MAGNETOM TrioTim syngo scanners. Note that we only use subjects who were scanned using MPRAGE sequence to minimize the effect of different scanning protocols. The T1-weighted images were acquired for 176 sagittal slices with the following parameters: repetition time (TR) = 2300 ms, echo time (TE) = 2.98 ms, flip angle = 9°, and voxel size = $1 \times 1 \times 1$ mm^3.

All the MR images were preprocessed by skull stripping [13], cerebellum removal, and tissue segmentation into white matter (WM), gray matter (GM), and cerebrospinal fluid (CSF) [14]. The anatomical automatic labeling (AAL) atlas [15], parcellated with 90 predefined regions, was registered using HAM-MER^2 [16,17] to the native space of each subject. We then computed WM, GM and CSF tissue volumes in each region and used them as features, *i.e.*, obtaining 90 WM, 90 GM and 90 CSF features, for each subject. 56 PD and 56 normal control (NC) subjects are used in our experiments.

To formulate the problem, we consider N training samples, each with a $d = 270$ dimensional feature vector. Let $\mathbf{X} \in \mathbb{R}^{N \times d}$ denote the training data, in which each row indicates a training sample, and $\mathbf{y} \in \mathbb{R}^N$ their corresponding labels. We seek to determine the labels for the test samples, $\mathbf{X}_{tst} \in \mathbb{R}^{N_{tst} \times d}$. After feature-sample selection, $\hat{N}$ samples and $\hat{d}$ features are selected, yielding to a new data matrix, $\hat{\mathbf{X}} \in \mathbb{R}^{\hat{N} \times \hat{d}}$, and train labels, $\hat{\mathbf{y}} \in \mathbb{R}^{\hat{N}}$, and same N_{tst} test samples but each with $\hat{d}$ features, $\hat{\mathbf{X}}_{tst} \in \mathbb{R}^{N_{tst} \times \hat{d}}$.^{3}

4   Joint Feature-Sample Selection (JFSS)

Selecting good features and samples is critical in building reliable machine learning models. This process not only improves the generalization capability of the learned model, but also speeds up the learning process. In many applications, it is a cumbersome task to acquire the best samples and features for a learning task. Particularly in our application, feature vectors extracted from MRI data are quite prone to noise. Many researches are conducted on feature and sample selection in the recent years [5,18–20], but few of them consider a joint formulation [21]. Feature selection and sample selection affect one another, and a separate selection might not lead to the best feature-sample subset, thus limiting the subsequent classification performance.

To this end, we aim to select only important samples and features to best describe a linear classification/regression model. In our method, we consider sparsity both in features and samples. The linear sparse regression model has been widely used for feature selection [18], where a sparse weight vector $\boldsymbol{\beta}$ is learned to best predict training labels. Accordingly, we are seeking to minimize

---

^{2} Could be downloaded at http://www.nitrc.org/projects/hammerwml.

^{3} Bold capital letters denote matrices (*e.g.*, $\mathbf{D}$). All non-bold letters denote scalar variables. d_{ij} denotes the scalar in the row i and column j of $\mathbf{D}$. $\|\mathbf{d}\|_2^2 = \langle \mathbf{d}, \mathbf{d} \rangle = \sum_i d_i^2$ denotes the squared Euclidean Norm of $\mathbf{d}$. $\|\mathbf{D}\|_*$ designates the nuclear norm (sum of singular values) of $\mathbf{D}$. $\|\mathbf{d}\|_1 = \sum_i |d_i|$ denotes the l_1 norm of the vector $\mathbf{d}$.

$\|\mathbf{y} - \mathbf{X}\boldsymbol{\beta}\|_2^2$ by keeping $\boldsymbol{\beta}$ sparse at the same time. Nevertheless, doing this separate from sample selection leads to a set of features which were affected by the noisy samples already present in the data. Instead, we jointly select features and samples when constructing a linear classification/regression model, which accounts for redundant data in both domains, simultaneously. Specifically, we introduce two vectors $\boldsymbol{\alpha}$ and $\boldsymbol{\beta}$, which are used to select samples and features, respectively. We impose a ℓ_1 regularization on both to ensure selection of the smallest subset in both domains. Joint feature-sample selection (JFSS) is thus performed by solving the following problem:

$$\min_{\boldsymbol{\alpha},\boldsymbol{\beta}} \ \|\hat{\boldsymbol{\alpha}}(\mathbf{y} - \mathbf{X}\boldsymbol{\beta})\|_2^2 + \lambda_1\|\boldsymbol{\alpha}\|_1 + \lambda_2\|\boldsymbol{\beta}\|_1, \quad \text{subject to } \hat{\boldsymbol{\alpha}} = \text{diag}(\boldsymbol{\alpha}). \tag{1}$$

The first term controls the overall data fitting error only for the selected samples indicated by $\boldsymbol{\alpha}$. The second and third terms are to ensure the selection of the smallest number of the most meaningful samples and features. To avoid the trivial solution for the optimization variable $\boldsymbol{\alpha}$, we further impose a condition so that at least a minimum number of the best representing samples will be selected. The iterative optimization procedure for optimizing $\boldsymbol{\alpha}$ discard the samples in each iteration. It is stopped, when the desired number of samples are selected. The number of the desired samples is determined through cross validation to avoid over-fitting. Some previous works have also used a common procedure to avoid trivial solutions [21, 22].

Solving the above problem is a cumbersome task, since the first term introduces a quadratic term. In order to solve problem (1), we break it down to two sub-problems and solve them iteratively. In each iteration, we optimize the objective by alternatively fixing one variable and optimizing for the other, until convergence. Specifically, optimizing for $\boldsymbol{\beta}$, while fixing $\boldsymbol{\alpha}$ and therefore $\hat{\boldsymbol{\alpha}}$, would reduce to:

$$\min_{\boldsymbol{\beta}} \ \|\hat{\boldsymbol{\alpha}}\mathbf{y} - \hat{\boldsymbol{\alpha}}\mathbf{X}\boldsymbol{\beta}\|_2^2 + \lambda_2\|\boldsymbol{\beta}\|_1. \tag{2}$$

Similarly, the optimization step for $\boldsymbol{\alpha}$, while fixing $\boldsymbol{\beta}$, would be:

$$\min_{\boldsymbol{\alpha}} \ \|\hat{\boldsymbol{\alpha}}(\mathbf{y} - \mathbf{X}\boldsymbol{\beta})\|_2^2 + \lambda_1\|\boldsymbol{\alpha}\|_1, \quad \text{subject to } \hat{\boldsymbol{\alpha}} = \text{diag}(\boldsymbol{\alpha}), \tag{3}$$

which is equivalent to solving:

$$\min_{\boldsymbol{\alpha}} \ \|(\mathbf{y} - \mathbf{X}\boldsymbol{\beta})^\top \boldsymbol{\alpha}\|_2^2 + \lambda_1\|\boldsymbol{\alpha}\|_1. \tag{4}$$

Both sub-problems could be optimized using an Alternating Direction Method of Multipliers (ADMM) [23].

It is noteworthy that the above procedure could also be used for classification. The first term learns a linear regression model with weights $\boldsymbol{\beta}$ to reconstruct $\mathbf{y}$ from $\mathbf{X}$, which could be used as a classification tool by discretizing the $\mathbf{y}$ values into classes. We add a single column of 1s to $\mathbf{X}$ (*i.e.*, $\mathbf{X} = [\mathbf{X} \ \mathbf{1}]$) to create a linear classifier model with a bias term. We use this classification scheme as a baseline method in the experiments referred to as Sparse Regression (SR).

5 Robust Classification (Robust LDA)

Even with selection of the most discriminative features and best samples, there might still be some noise present in the data. These noise elements of data can adversely influence the classifier learning process. Therefore, we further model the noise in the features matrix, $\mathbf{X}$. In other words, after discarding some samples and features using our JFSS, we account for the intra-sample outliers (noises in feature values) in $\hat{\mathbf{X}}$ to further reduce the influences of noise elements in the data. For this purpose, following [24,25], we assume that the data matrix $\hat{\mathbf{X}}$ could be spanned on a low-rank subspace and therefore should be rank-deficient. This assumption supports the fact that samples from same classes should be more correlated [11,25]. In order to achieve a robust classifier, we use a same idea as in [11], which was proposed for robust regression. In our case, classification is posed as a binary regression problem, in which a transform $\mathbf{w}$ maps each sample in $\hat{\mathbf{X}}$ to a binary label in $\mathbf{y}$. In the linear case, this could be modeled with a Linear Discriminant Analysis (LDA), which learns a linear mapping to minimize the intra-class discrimination and maximize the inter-class variation. Furthermore, LS-LDA [10] models the LDA problem in a least-squares formulation: $\min_{\mathbf{w}} \|\hat{\mathbf{y}} - \hat{\mathbf{X}}\mathbf{w}\|_2^2$, where $\mathbf{w}$ is a projection of $\hat{\mathbf{X}}$ to the space of labels, $\hat{\mathbf{y}}$.

Assume $\hat{\mathbf{X}}$ is the data matrix corrupted by noise. Therefore, we can say $\hat{\mathbf{X}} = \hat{\mathbf{D}} + \mathbf{E}$, where $\hat{\mathbf{D}} \in \mathbb{R}^{\hat{N} \times \hat{d}}$ is the underlying noise-free component and $\mathbf{E} \in \mathbb{R}^{\hat{N} \times \hat{d}}$ is the noise component. To model this noise in the above formulation and learn the mapping $\mathbf{w}$ from the clean data $\hat{\mathbf{D}}$, we utilize the scenario in [11] and rewrite our problem as:

$$\min_{\mathbf{w}, \mathbf{D}, \mathbf{E}} \frac{\eta}{2} \|\hat{\mathbf{y}} - \mathbf{D}\mathbf{w}\|_2^2 + \|\hat{\mathbf{D}}\|_* + \gamma \|\mathbf{E}\|_1, \quad \text{subject to } \hat{\mathbf{X}} = \hat{\mathbf{D}} + \mathbf{E}, \mathbf{D} = [\hat{\mathbf{D}} \ 1],$$

(5)

where the first term learns the mapping $\mathbf{w}$ from the clean data and projects the samples to the label space. The second and the third terms guarantee the rank-deficiency of the data matrix $\hat{\mathbf{D}}$ and also $\mathbf{E}$ to be sparse, respectively. These two terms are similar to the Robust Principle Component Analysis (RPCA) [26]. RPCA is an unsupervised method, while the above formulation cleans the data in a supervised manner. Particularly, the matrix $\hat{\mathbf{D}}$ retains the subspace of $\hat{\mathbf{X}}$, which is most correlated to the labels $\hat{\mathbf{y}}$. The solution to problem (5) could be achieved by writing the Lagrangian function and iteratively solving for $\mathbf{w}, \mathbf{D}, \hat{\mathbf{D}}$ and $\mathbf{E}$ one at a time, while fixing others [11].

In most cases, due to the presence of noise in the test data, the classification accuracy may drop dramatically in the testing phase. For cleaning the test data, one can use RPCA [26], but again it is unsupervised. To this end, we utilize our data cleaned in, $\hat{\mathbf{D}}$. We de-noise the test data, $\hat{\mathbf{X}}_{tst}$, by representing them as a combination of the training data: $\hat{\mathbf{D}}_{tst} = \hat{\mathbf{D}}\mathbf{Z}_{tst}$, where $\mathbf{Z}_{tst}$ is the coefficient matrix for the combination. To clean the data, we model the combination as: $\hat{\mathbf{X}}_{tst} = \hat{\mathbf{D}}\mathbf{Z}_{tst} + \mathbf{E}_{tst}$, where $\mathbf{E}_{tst} \in \mathbb{R}^{N_{tst} \times \hat{d}}$ is the noise component of the test data. In order for the linear combination to be locally compact, we further impose the low-rank constraint on the coefficients, as in [24,27]:

$$\min_{\mathbf{Z}_{tst}, \hat{\mathbf{E}}_{tst}} \quad \|\mathbf{Z}_{tst}\|_* + \lambda \|\mathbf{E}_{tst}\|_1, \quad \text{subject to } \hat{\mathbf{X}}_{tst} = \hat{\mathbf{D}} \mathbf{Z}_{tst} + \mathbf{E}_{tst}. \tag{6}$$

This optimization problem could be solved using linearized ALM method as in [27]. After cleaning the test data, the prediction for the classification output is calculated as $\mathbf{y}_{tst} = [\hat{\mathbf{D}} \mathbf{Z}_{tst} \ \mathbf{1}] \mathbf{w}$. Same as in LS-LDA, $\mathbf{y}_{tst}$ is used as the decision value and the binary class labels are produced using the k-nearest neighbor method.

6   Experiments

In order to evaluate the proposed approach, we set up experiments on both synthetic and PPMI datasets. Baseline classifiers under comparison include linear support vector machines (SVM), sparse regression (SR), as described in Sect. 4, and the original LS-LDA [10]. To evaluate the JFSS procedure, we compare the results with separate feature and sample selections (FSS), sparse feature selection (SFS) and no feature sample selection (no FSS). Furthermore, we report results using other prominent methods for feature transforms like min-redundancy max-relevance (mRMR) [20] and principle component analysis (PCA). The results for the baseline methods were generated using 10-fold cross validation and best parameters for each of them were selected (like ours).

Synthetic Data: We construct two independent subspaces of dimensionality 100 (as described in [24]), and sample 500 samples from each subspace. This leads to a binary classification problem. We gradually add additional noisy samples and features to the data and evaluate the proposed JFSS and robust classification schemes using this data. Figure 2 shows the mean accuracy results of

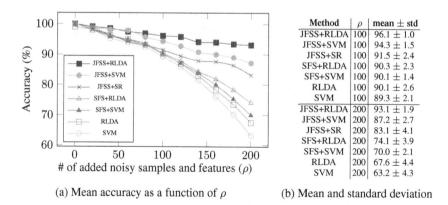

(a) Mean accuracy as a function of ρ

Method	ρ	mean $\pm$ std
JFSS+RLDA	100	96.1 $\pm$ 1.0
JFSS+SVM	100	94.3 $\pm$ 1.5
JFSS+SR	100	91.5 $\pm$ 2.4
SFS+RLDA	100	90.3 $\pm$ 2.3
SFS+SVM	100	90.1 $\pm$ 1.4
RLDA	100	90.1 $\pm$ 2.6
SVM	100	89.3 $\pm$ 2.1
JFSS+RLDA	200	93.1 $\pm$ 1.9
JFSS+SVM	200	87.2 $\pm$ 2.7
JFSS+SR	200	83.1 $\pm$ 4.1
SFS+RLDA	200	74.1 $\pm$ 3.9
SFS+SVM	200	70.0 $\pm$ 2.1
RLDA	200	67.6 $\pm$ 4.4
SVM	200	63.2 $\pm$ 4.3

(b) Mean and standard deviation

Fig. 2. Results comparisons on synthetic data, for three different runs.

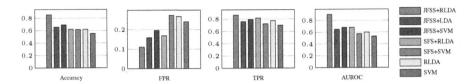

Fig. 3. Comparisons of results by the proposed (JFSS + RLDA) and the baseline methods. (Color figure online)

three different runs as a function of the additional number of noisy features and samples, with a 10-fold cross-validation strategy. Our JFSS coupled with the classifiers is able to select better subset of features and samples for improved results. Furthermore, it acts more robustly against the increase of noise elements. This is attributed to the de-noising process introduced by our RLDA.

PPMI Data: The details of the data are described in Sect. 3. For quantitative evaluations, the accuracy, true positive rate (TPR), false positive rate (FPR) and area under ROC are calculated and are shown in Fig. 3, in comparisons with the baseline methods. The combination of JFSS and RLDA is outperforming all other methods by a significant margin. Table 1 also shows the diagnosis accuracy of the proposed technique (RLDA + JFSS) in comparisons with different feature/sample selection/transform methods, using a 10-fold cross-validation strategy. The optimization parameters are all chosen by a grid search for best performance using the same cross-validation strategy on training data. The proposed method outperforms all others. This could be because the data has many redundant samples and features and also suffers from noise corruption, and we deal with both issues properly.

Discussions: Due to the huge amount of noise in the original data and redundant features and samples, we introduced JFSS framework to select the best subsets of both sample and feature spaces. Even with JFSS, portions of noise elements still exists in the data, which we de-noise using RLDA. On the other hand, RLDA alone does not provide good performance, since the amount of noisy and irrelevant feature values are high in the data. RLDA and in general most

Table 1. Accuracy results of the PD/NC classification, compared to the baseline classifiers and different feature-sample selection/transform techniques.

Classifier	Selection/transform method					
	JFSS	FSS	SFS	no FSS	mRMR	PCA
Robust LDA	**82.5**	78.1	72.5	61.9	70.8	65.5
LDA	65.5	62.5	62.2	56.6	62.1	57.0
SVM	69.1	62.4	61.5	55.2	59.8	58.0
SR	65.1	61.8	59.3	–	–	–

robust machine learning methods can deal with a controlled amount of noise, since they assume a sparse noise element in the data (with ℓ_1 regularization). Using JFSS, we discard a huge amount of redundant data, and RLDA is then utilized to de-noise the remaining, while classifying the data.

Furthermore, as confirmed by the results, we could distinguish PD from NC using only MRI. With the progression of PD, patients' brains are affected heavily through time. So, these data-driven methods could be of great use for early diagnosis, or prediction of the disease progression.

7 Conclusions

In this paper, we have introduced a joint feature-sample selection (JFSS) framework along with a robust classification approach for PD diagnosis. We have established robustness in both training and testing phases. We verified our method using subjects excerpted from the PPMI dataset, a first large-scale longitudinal study of PD. Our method outperforms several baseline methods on both synthetic data and the PD/NC classification problem. As a direction for future works, one can use clinical scores and other imaging modalities to predict the PD progress in subjects, or to improve the accuracy. More effective features can also be extracted to further improve the diagnosis accuracy.

References

1. Ziegler, D.A., Augustinack, J.C.: Harnessing advances in structural MRI to enhance research on Parkinson's disease. Imaging Med. **5**(2), 91–94 (2013)
2. Braak, H., Tredici, K., Rub, U., de Vos, R., Steur, E.J., Braak, E.: Staging of brain pathology related to sporadic Parkinsons disease. Neurobiol. Aging **24**(2), 197–211 (2003)
3. Duchesne, S., Rolland, Y., Varin, M.: Automated computer differential classification in parkinsonian syndromes via pattern analysis on MRI. Acad. Radiol. **16**(1), 61–70 (2009)
4. Prashanth, R., Roy, S.D., Mandal, P.K., Ghosh, S.: Automatic classification and prediction models for early Parkinson's disease diagnosis from SPECT imaging. Expert Syst. Appl. **41**(7), 3333–3342 (2014)
5. Thung, K.H., Wee, C.Y., Yap, P.T., Shen, D.: Neurodegenerative disease diagnosis using incomplete multi-modality data via matrix shrinkage and completion. NeuroImage **91**, 386–400 (2014)
6. Bron, E., Smits, M., van Swieten, J., Niessen, W., Klein, S.: Feature selection based on SVM significance maps for classification of dementia. In: Wu, G., Zhang, D., Zhou, L. (eds.) MLMI 2014. LNCS, vol. 8679, pp. 272–279. Springer, Heidelberg (2014)
7. Oh, J.H., Kim, Y.B., Gurnani, P., Rosenblatt, K., Gao, J.: Biomarker selection for predicting alzheimer disease using high-resolution MALDI-TOF data. In: IEEE International Conference on Bioinformatics and Bioengineering, pp. 464–471, October 2007

8. Rohlfing, T., Brandt, R., Menzel, R., Maurer, C.R.: Evaluation of atlas selection strategies for atlas-based image segmentation with application to confocal microscopy images of bee brains. NeuroImage **21**(4), 1428–1442 (2004)
9. Cormen, T.H., Leiserson, C.E., Rivest, R.L., Stein, C.: Introduction to Algorithms, 3rd edn. The MIT Press, Cambridge (2009)
10. De la Torre, F.: A least-squares framework for component analysis. IEEE Trans. Pattern Anal. Mach. Intell. **34**(6), 1041–1055 (2012)
11. Huang, D., Cabral, R., De la Torre, F.: Robust regression. In: European Conference on Computer Vision, pp. 616–630 (2012)
12. Marek, K., et al.: The Parkinson progression marker initiative (PPMI). Prog. Neurobiol. **95**(4), 629–635 (2011)
13. Wang, Y., Nie, J., Yap, P.T., Li, G., Shi, F., Geng, X., Guo, L., Shen, D.: Knowledge-guided robust MRI brain extraction for diverse large-scale neuroimaging studies on humans and non-human primates. PLOS ONE **9**(1), e77810 (2014)
14. Lim, K., Pfefferbaum, A.: Segmentation of MR brain images into cerebrospinal fluid spaces, white and gray matter. J. Comput. Assist. Tomogr. **13**, 588–593 (1989)
15. Tzourio-Mazoyer, N., et al.: Automated anatomical labeling of activations in SPM using a macroscopic anatomical parcellation of the MNI MRI single-subject brain. NeuroImage **15**(1), 273–289 (2002)
16. Shen, D., Davatzikos, C.: HAMMER: hierarchical attribute matching mechanism for elastic registration. IEEE Trans. Med. Imaging **21**, 1421–1439 (2002)
17. Wang, Y., Nie, J., Yap, P.-T., Shi, F., Guo, L., Shen, D.: Robust deformable-surface-based skull-stripping for large-scale studies. In: Fichtinger, G., Martel, A., Peters, T. (eds.) MICCAI 2011, Part III. LNCS, vol. 6893, pp. 635–642. Springer, Heidelberg (2011)
18. Nie, F., Huang, H., Cai, X., Ding, C.H.: Efficient and robust feature selection via joint $\ell_{2,1}$-norms minimization. In: Neural Information Processing Systems, pp. 1813–1821 (2010)
19. Coates, A., Lee, H., Ng, A.: An analysis of single-layer networks in unsupervised feature learning. In: AI and STAT, JMLR, vol. 15, pp. 215–223 (2011)
20. Peng, H., Long, F., Ding, C.: Feature selection based on mutual information criteria of max-dependency, max-relevance, and min-redundancy. IEEE Trans. Pattern Anal. Mach. Intell. **27**(8), 1226–1238 (2005)
21. Mohsenzadeh, Y., et al.: The relevance sample-feature machine: a sparse Bayesian learning approach to joint feature-sample selection. IEEE Trans. Cybern. **43**(6), 2241–2254 (2013)
22. Argyriou, A., Evgeniou, T., Pontil, M.: Multi-task feature learning. In: Neural Information Processing Systems, pp. 41–48 (2007)
23. Boyd, S., et al.: Distributed optimization and statistical learning via the alternating direction method of multipliers. Found. Trends Mach. Learn. **3**(1), 1–122 (2011)
24. Liu, G., Lin, Z., Yan, S., Sun, J., Yu, Y., Ma, Y.: Robust recovery of subspace structures by low-rank representation. IEEE Trans. Pattern Anal. Mach. Intell. **35**(1), 171–184 (2013)
25. Goldberg, A.B., Zhu, X., Recht, B., Xu, J.M., Nowak, R.D.: Transduction with matrix completion: three birds with one stone. In: Neural Information Processing Systems, pp. 757–765 (2010)
26. Candès, E.J., Li, X., Ma, Y., Wright, J.: Robust principal component analysis. J. ACM **58**(3), 11:1–11:37 (2011)
27. Lin, Z., Liu, R., Su, Z.: Linearized alternating direction method with adaptive penalty for low-rank representation. In: Neural Information Processing Systems, pp. 612–620 (2011)

Dynamic Tree-Based Large-Deformation Image Registration for Multi-atlas Segmentation

Pei Zhang, Guorong Wu, Yaozong Gao, Pew-Thian Yap,
and Dinggang Shen$^{(\boxtimes)}$

Department of Radiology, Biomedical Research Imaging Center (BRIC),
The University of North Carolina at Chapel Hill, Chapel Hill, USA
dinggang_shen@med.unc.edu

Abstract. Multi-atlas segmentation is a powerful approach to automated anatomy delineation via fusing label information from a set of spatially normalized atlases. For simplicity, many existing methods perform pairwise image registration, leading to inaccurate segmentation especially when shape variation is large. In this paper, we propose a dynamic tree-based strategy for effective large-deformation registration and multi-atlas segmentation. To deal with local minima caused by large shape variation, coarse estimates of deformations are first obtained via alignment of automatically localized landmark points. A dynamic tree capturing the structural relationships between images is then used to further reduce misalignment errors. Validation on two real human brain datasets, ADNI and LPBA40, shows that our method significantly improves registration and segmentation accuracy.

1 Introduction

Multi-atlas segmentation is an automated approach to delineating anatomical structures of a target image by borrowing complementary information from multiple pre-annotated atlases. Segmentation labels from multiple atlases that are registered to the target image are combined to obtain the ultimate segmentation result. This approach avoids not only time-consuming manual annotation but also potential bias introduced by segmentation with only one single atlas. Due to its promising results, it has been widely used in medical image analysis to segment the brain [1], the heart [2] and abdominal organs [11].

Although much effort has been put to improve the accuracy of label fusion, much less emphasis has been put on image registration. Most of the existing multi-atlas segmentation methods merely perform simple pairwise registration [1,2] by aligning each atlas independently to the target image. This approach fails to consider the correlation between atlases and thus leads to inconsistency among the atlases when labeling the same anatomical structure. Simple pairwise

D. Shen—This work was supported in part by a UNC BRIC-Radiology start-up fund, and NIH grants (EB006733, EB008374, EB009634, MH088520 and NIHM 5R01MH091645-02).

© Springer International Publishing Switzerland 2016
B. Menze et al. (Eds.): MCV Workshop 2015, LNCS 9601, pp. 137–145, 2016.
DOI: 10.1007/978-3-319-42016-5_13

registration also does not take advantage of the structural similarity between images to help overcome registration related problems such as local minima. Such problem occurs quite often when images from different populations (i.e., patients and healthy controls) vary dramatically in anatomical structures.

There have been some recent attempts to overcome the above problems by using more sophisticated registration strategies. For example, Hoang Duc et al.[5] attempted to establish the relationship across atlases and the target image by iteratively registering them to an evolving group mean image [8]. However, this only works well when images in the group can be registered reasonably well. Also, the mean image is sensitive to registration outliers and may be unstable in case of large shape variation. A better approach described in [7] links images according to their similarity using a tree structure and performs a series of registration of adjacent images. This breaks down the complex registration process into a number of simpler ones and helps reduce local minima.

In this paper we describe a registration scheme for multi-atlas segmentation under large deformation. Similar to [7], a tree structure is used for robust registration. The registration outcome is then applied for multi-atlas segmentation of either a single image or a group of images. Our work differs from [7] in three major aspects. *First*, images with similar intensity values are not necessarily similar in anatomy. Hence, in contrast to [7] we propose to construct the tree using shape similarity evaluated based on the closeness of landmark points localized at structure boundaries in different images. *Second*, unlike the affine initialization used in [7], we use the localized landmark points to initialize image registration. Good initialization has been shown to significantly improve registration accuracy, particularly when dealing with large shape variation [13]. *Finally*, we propose to utilize a dynamically updated tree, as opposed to the fixed one used in [7]. This is to ensure connections between images to be progressively refined to reduce misalignment.

2   Methodology

Our goal is to label one or more target images using a set of atlases, each with an intensity image and a segmentation image obtained by manual labeling of some regions of interest (ROIs). Note that each target image only has the intensity image. To simultaneously warp all atlases and target images to a common space for consistent segmentation, we perform the following steps: (1) seek corresponding landmark points among atlases and target images (Sect. 2.1); (2) perform initial registration using an initial tree generated by connecting all images using the landmark points (Sect. 2.2); (3) iteratively update the tree and registration results (Sect. 2.3). Label fusion can then be carried out for segmentation of the target images using the registered atlases. Each step is described in detail below.

2.1   Localization of Corresponding Landmark Points

We follow the method in [4] to detect landmark points on an image. A set of landmark points is first generated for each atlas in a semi-supervised manner.

These points, together with the atlases, are then used to train a set of point detectors, one for each landmark, using regression forests [3]. For a target image, each trained detector is then applied for landmark localization. Below we briefly describe each step (see [4] for details).

To generate the landmark points for each atlas, we randomly choose one atlas as the reference, generate a number of salient points on the reference by excluding flat regions, and propagate the points to the other atlases via non-rigid registration of segmentation images. Examples of the generated landmark points are shown in Fig. 1.

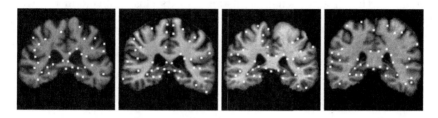

Fig. 1. Examples of the generated landmark points. Note that some landmarks reside in different slices and might not be visible.

By using the landmarks in the atlases, we train a detector for each landmark to predict its position from Haar-like image features of nearby voxel neighborhoods. We systematically sample a number of voxels around each landmark and record their displacements to the landmark together with the Haar-like features of their neighborhoods. Repeating this process for the corresponding landmarks in the other atlases leads to a set of displacement-feature pairs that can be used to train the detector to predict the displacement of the landmark from the each voxel based on the Haar features of its neighborhood. To learn such highly non-linear relationship, we use the regression forest [3], which consists of a collection of binary decision trees, each trained individually using a random subset of displacement-feature pairs.

To predict the displacement associated with a voxel, the corresponding features are passed through each tree of a detector until it reaches a leaf node of the tree. A "point jumping" technique and a multi-resolution strategy are then used for robust prediction (see [4] for details).

2.2   Tree Construction and Initial Registration

Once the landmark points for all atlases and target images have been localized, we use them to build a tree connecting images that are similar in anatomy for initial registration. Based on [7], we utilize the atlases to build a tree, onto which each target image is progressively attached. This helps avoid having to run the registration again whenever a new image needs to be segmented.

An adjacency matrix is first generated based on the Euclidean distance between the corresponding landmark points of each pair of atlases. Based on the adjacency matrix, a minimum spanning tree is then generated using Prim's algorithm. Each edge of the tree connects a pair of atlases and encodes their distance. In the tree, any pair of atlases is connected by a unique path (i.e., a set of edges). An atlas with the least sum of distances to all other atlases is chosen as the root of the tree. This root is fixed throughout the whole registration process. The target images are then progressively appended to the tree by recursively attaching each to its closest atlas or target image in tree. Each time when the tree is updated using this process, among all target images, only the target image that has the smallest distance to its closest image in the tree is attached.

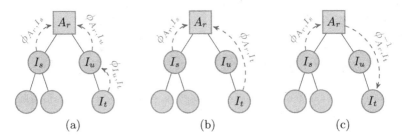

Fig. 2. Registration of one image (I_s) to another (I_t) via the root node (A_r): (a) Register adjacent images along the respective paths from I_s and I_t to root A_r; (b) Concatenate the deformation fields along the paths, i.e., $\phi_{A_r,I_t} = \phi_{I_u,I_t} \circ \phi_{A_r,I_u}$; (c) Concatenate the inverse of ϕ_{A_r,I_t} and with ϕ_{A_r,I_s} to obtain the final deformation field from I_s to I_t.

Once the tree is built, registration between a pair of images in the tree can be achieved using the root atlas A_r as the bridge (Fig. 2). Specifically, we use the following steps to warp an image I_s to another image I_t: (1) determine the path that connects I_s and A_r; (2) perform pairwise registration between adjacent images along this path from I_s to A_r; (3) concatenate the resulting deformation fields to obtain the deformation field from I_s to A_r, denoted as ϕ_{A_r,I_s}; (4) repeat the above three steps to obtain the deformation field from I_t to A_r, denoted as ϕ_{A_r,I_t}; (5) estimate the inverse of ϕ_{A_r,I_t}, denoted as ϕ_{A_r,I_t}^{-1}; (6) compute the deformation field from I_s to I_t, ϕ_{I_t,I_s}, by concatenating ϕ_{A_r,I_s} and ϕ_{A_r,I_t}^{-1}, i.e., $\phi_{I_t,I_s} = \phi_{A_r,I_s} \circ \phi_{A_r,I_t}^{-1}$, where $\circ$ is the composition operator. In the current work, registration between adjacent images is performed using diffeomorphic Demons [10].

The above process is repeated to register all atlases to each target image. The resulting deformation fields are then used to warp the segmentation images associated with the atlases to target images for segmentation via label fusion.

Although we use corresponding landmark points to encourage connections between images of similar anatomy in the initial tree construction, some target images may be still inappropriately connected to the tree due to the simple

Euclidean distance for similarity, thus introducing more local minima to registration. This is especially the case when registering images under large deformation. To reduce local minima caused by large shape variation, here we propose two solutions: one is to initialize the registration with the corresponding points, which can be achieved by thin-plate spline (TPS) interpolation, and the other is reconnect target images that are inappropriately connected, which will be detailed below.

2.3   Iterative Registration with Dynamic Tree

We introduce a feed back loop after initial registration to reconnect poorly connected target images. Hence the tree is dynamically updated to refine registration.

To determine the appropriateness of the connection of a target image to the tree, we warp the landmark points on an atlas onto the target image and average the distances between all warped points and their corresponding counterparts on the target image. We repeat this process for all atlases and finally obtain an overall average landmark distance that can be used to tell how well the given target image is connected to the tree. A smaller overall distance indicates better connection.

As the landmark points only cover the brain sparsely, the above metric merely gives a coarse indication of the appropriateness of the connection. For more localized sensitivity, we also (1) warp the segmentation images of the atlases onto the target image, (2) estimate a segmentation image for the target image using the set of warped segmentation images based on [7], (3) warp the resulting segmentation image back onto each atlas, and (4) compute the Dice ratio between the segmentation image of each atlas and the warped segmentation image of the target image. We use the overall Dice ratio, computed by averaging the ratios across ROIs and atlases, as another metric for evaluation of connection appropriateness. This segmentation-based metric is combined with the above landmark-based metric via weighted averaging to form a combined metric after normalizing both to have a zero mean and a unit variance.

Once we have computed the connection appropriateness of each target image, we can select a subset of target images with the best connections to the tree. This can be achieved by ranking all the target images by the appropriateness and choosing the top ones. Let $\mathcal{A}$ be the set of atlases, $\mathcal{U}$ the selected subset of target images, and $\mathcal{T}$ the rest of the target images. We repeat the following steps until $\mathcal{T} = \emptyset$ or no new tree can be generated:

(1) Rebuild the connections of the images in $\mathcal{T}$ to the tree by recursive attachment as described in Sect. 2.2. Note that the images in $\mathcal{U}$ are treated as atlases and their links to the tree will not be changed in this process. The combined metric instead of the landmark distance is used to guide the reattachment process;

(2) Run registration with the new tree. As the images in $\mathcal{U}$ are well linked to the tree, the deformation fields between those images and atlases are likely to be reliably estimated. Hence, we can use these deformation fields to guide

the registration between a pair of images, I_s and I_t, as follows (Fig. 3): (i) find its most recent ancestor node in $\mathcal{A} \cup \mathcal{U}$ for target image $I_t \in \mathcal{T}$; (ii) estimate the deformation field from the ancestor to I_t; (iii) concatenate the resulting deformation field with that from I_s to the ancestor; (iv) use the composite deformation field to initialize the registration from I_s to I_t;

(3) Extend $\mathcal{U}$ by adding the images in $\mathcal{T}$ whose connection appropriateness improves after registration. If not enough images are added, we rank all images in $\mathcal{T}$ by the connection appropriateness and choose the top ones as before. This is to ensure that the whole registration completes in a few iterations for efficiency. We require at least a fixed portion (i.e., 10 %) of the targeted images to be added to $\mathcal{U}$ at each iteration.

3   Experiments

We demonstrate the efficacy of our method on two real datasets: the ADNI dataset[1] and the LPBA40 dataset [9]. For each dataset, FLIRT [6] was used to align all the images via affine transform to a common space before all subsequent experiments.

The segmentation images in the two datasets were used for evaluation. Segmentation of the LPBA40 dataset was carried out by experts. Only 54 out of the 56 labels were used for evaluation, excluding the cerebellum and the brainstem. Segmentation of the ADNI dataset into gray matter (GM), white matter (WM), cerebrospinal fluid (CSF) and ventricle (VN) was done using FAST [14].

Each point detector was trained at 4 different image resolutions, at each of which 10 trees were trained, amounting to a total of 40 trees. To train a detector, we sampled 6000 voxels around the landmark point and computed their Haar-like features based on the intensity image of each atlas. For each tree, the maximum depth was set to 12 and the input of each leaf node was required to be at least 10 sampled voxels.

We compared our method with the method proposed by [7] (MABMIS for short), which builds a fixed tree based on image intensity difference to guide the registration for multi-atlas segmentation. The code is available at http://www.nitrc.org/projects/mabmis. The comparison is to show the advantage of the use of shape similarity for tree construction, corresponding landmark points for initialization of image registration, and the dynamic tree registration scheme. We computed the Dice ratio of the segmentation image of each target image with respect to the segmentation image of each atlas after warping to the space of the target image. Averaging the Dice ratios across atlases for each target image and then across target images leads to an overall Dice ratio that was used for quantitative evaluation of the methods.

3.1   ADNI Dataset

We randomly selected 150 baseline images from the dataset: 50 from healthy controls, 50 from mild cognitive impairment patients and 50 from Alzheimer's

---

[1] http://adni.loni.usc.edu/.

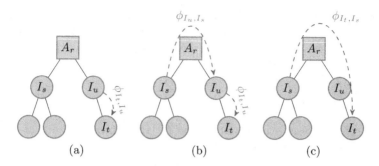

Fig. 3. Registration of one image (I_s) to another (I_t) via the help of images in $\mathcal{A} \cup \mathcal{U}$: (a) Register its most recent ancestor, $I_u \in \mathcal{A} \cup \mathcal{U}$, to image I_t; (b) Concatenate the resulting deformation field ϕ_{I_t,I_u} with the deformation field from I_s to I_u, ϕ_{I_u,I_s}; (c) Initialize the registration from I_s to I_t with the composite deformation field.

Table 1. Overall Dice ratios for different tree-based image registration methods.

Methods	CSF	VN	GM	WM
i-Tree	61.6 %	87.3 %	61.4 %	75.0 %
p-Tree	62.0 %	87.6 %	61.7 %	75.4 %
p-Tree+TPS	62.7 %	87.9 %	62.2 %	76.2 %
Dynamic tree	63.7 %	88.1 %	63.2 %	77.2 %

disease patients. All of the selected images were then preprocessed using the following steps: (1) Anterior commissure/posterior commissure alignment correction; (2) Inhomogeneity correction using the N3 algorithm; (3) Skull stripping using Brain Surface Extractor and Brain Extraction Tool; (4) Intensity normalization via histogram matching.

We randomly chose 10 images from each group as the atlases and used the rest as the target images that need to be segmented, leading to 30 atlases and 120 target images. Using an atlas as the reference, we generated over 500 landmark points covering the whole brain and propagated them to other atlases. The landmark detectors, trained using these landmark points, were applied to localize landmark points in each target image.

The landmark points were used to build a "point" tree (p-Tree) and based on this tree the images were registered as described in Sect. 2.2. To demonstrate the effectiveness of the p-Tree in image registration, we built an "intensity" tree (i-Tree) using the intensity differences between images, as in MABMIS. The overall Dice ratios shown in Table 1 indicate that, compared with the i-Tree, the p-Tree gives better registration accuracy.

Table 1 also shows that when a TPS fitting of the landmark points is used for initializing the deformation in the diffeomorphic Demons algorithm, registration accuracy can be remarkably improved. Further improvements can be obtain using the p-Tree with the dynamic tree registration strategy described in Sect. 2.3. The improvement given by the dynamic tree based method is statistically significant (two-tailed t-test, $p < 0.01$) when compared with each of the other methods. For example, the improvement is 0.8 %, 1.8 % and 2.2 % within the VN, GM and WM compared with the MABMIS method.

3.2   LPBA40 Dataset

We repeated the above experiment on the LPBA40 dataset. 8 out of the total 40 images were used as atlases for the same atlas and target ratio as used in Sect. 3.1. Due to the limit of space, we only summarize the results here without showing the detailed figures.

Experimental results show that the p-Tree+TPS works similarly or significantly better than the i-Tree within most of ROIs. In fact, the accuracy is increased by more than 1 % for 29 out of 54 ROIs, with the largest improvement given by the left postcentral gyrus (5.6 %). The accuracy is further improved by the dynamic tree based strategy, leading to over 1 % improvement within 26 out of 54 ROIs compared with the p-Tree+TPS. The maximum improvement is given by the right postcentral gyrus (2.4 %). Averaging the overall Dice ratios over all 54 ROIs leads to 67.4 %, 68.6 %, and 69.6 %, respectively, for the i-Tree, p-Tree+TPS and dynamic tree based strategy.

We further demonstrate the advantages of our method using multi-atlas segmentation with the sparse patch based label fusion method described in [12]. The results show that our method gives significant improvement over the i-Tree. For example, the p-Tree+TPS leads to 27 out of 54 ROIs with more than 1 % improvement in segmentation accuracy. The maximum improvement is found in the left postcentral gyrus (3.3 %). The segmentation accuracy is further improved by the dynamic tree based scheme, with more than 1 % improvement for 22 out of 54 ROIs, compared with the p-Tree+TPS. The left cuneus gives the largest improvement (3.4 %). The averaged overall Dice ratios for the i-Tree, p-Tree+TPS and dynamic tree based strategy are 73.0 %, 73.8 % and 74.7 %.

4   Conclusions and Future Work

We have described a method that can accurately register a set of atlases to a set of target images for multi-atlas segmentation. Our method deals with large-deformation registration by using landmark points in a dynamic tree-based image registration strategy. Local minima caused by large shape variation can be avoided by encouraging registration between images with comparable anatomy, by good registration initialization, and by dynamically reconnection of images to the tree.

Experiments show that our method is able to achieve good results on two real datasets. We show that our method is superior to a tree based image registration [7]. It can not only further improve registration accuracy, but also greatly help label fusion for better segmentation. This clearly demonstrates the importance of accurate image registration for multi-atlas segmentation. In the future, we will investigate a more advanced approach to using the landmark points for tree construction and registration initialization.

References

1. Asman, A.J., Landman, B.A.: Non-local statistical label fusion for multi-atlas segmentation. Med. Image Anal. **17**(2), 194–208 (2013)
2. Bai, W., Shi, W., Ledig, C., Rueckert, D.: Multi-atlas segmentation with augmented features for cardiac MR images. Med. Image Anal. **19**(1), 98–109 (2015)
3. Criminisi, A., Shotton, J., Konukoglu, E.: Decision forests: a unified framework for classification, regression, density estimation, manifold learning and semi-supervised learning. Found. Trends® Comput. Graph. Vis. **7**(2–3), 81–227 (2012)
4. Han, D., Gao, Y., Wu, G., Yap, P.-T., Shen, D.: Robust anatomical landmark detection for MR brain image registration. In: Golland, P., Hata, N., Barillot, C., Hornegger, J., Howe, R. (eds.) MICCAI 2014, Part I. LNCS, vol. 8673, pp. 186–193. Springer, Heidelberg (2014)
5. Hoang Duc, A.K., Modat, M., Leung, K.K., Cardoso, M.J., Barnes, J., Kadir, T., Ourselin, S.: Using manifold learning for atlas selection in multi-atlas segmentation. PLoS ONE **8**(8), e70059 (2013)
6. Jenkinson, M., Smith, S.: A global optimisation method for robust affine registration of brain images. Med. Image Anal. **5**(2), 143–156 (2001)
7. Jia, H., Yap, P.T., Shen, D.: Iterative multi-atlas-based multi-image segmentation with tree-based registration. NeuroImage **59**(1), 422–430 (2012)
8. Rohlfing, T., Brandt, R., Menzel, R., Maurer, C.R.: Evaluation of atlas selection strategies for atlas-based image segmentation with application to confocal microscopy images of bee brains. NeuroImage **21**(4), 1428–1442 (2004)
9. Shattuck, D.W., Mirza, M., Adisetiyo, V., Hojatkashani, C., Salamon, G., Narr, K.L., Poldrack, R.A., Bilder, R.M., Toga, A.W.: Construction of a 3D probabilistic atlas of human cortical structures. NeuroImage **39**(3), 1064–1080 (2008)
10. Vercauteren, T., Pennec, X., Perchant, A., Ayache, N.: Diffeomorphic demons: efficient non-parametric image registration. NeuroImage **45**(Supplement 1), 61–72 (2009)
11. Wolz, R., Chu, C., Misawa, K., Fujiwara, M., Mori, K., Rueckert, D.: Automated abdominal multi-organ segmentation with subject-specific atlas generation. IEEE Trans. Med. Imaging **32**(9), 1723–1730 (2013)
12. Zhang, D., Guo, Q., Wu, G., Shen, D.: Sparse patch-based label fusion for multi-atlas segmentation. In: Yap, P.-T., Liu, T., Shen, D., Westin, C.-F., Shen, L. (eds.) MBIA 2012. LNCS, vol. 7509, pp. 94–102. Springer, Heidelberg (2012)
13. Zhang, P., Cootes, T.F.: Automatic construction of parts+geometry models for initialising groupwise registration. IEEE Trans. Med. Imaging **31**(2), 341–358 (2012)
14. Zhang, Y., Brady, M., Smith, S.: Segmentation of brain MR images through a hidden Markov random field model and the expectation-maximization algorithm. IEEE Trans. Med. Imaging **20**(1), 45–57 (2001)

Hippocampus Segmentation from MR Infant Brain Images via Boundary Regression

Yeqin Shao[1,2], Yanrong Guo[2], Yaozong Gao[2,3], Xin Yang[4],
and Dinggang Shen[2(✉)]

[1] Nantong University, Jiangsu 226019, China
[2] Department of Radiology and BRIC, University of North Carolina at Chapel
Hill, Chapel Hill, NC 27599, USA
dgshen@med.unc.edu
[3] Department of Computer Science, University of North Carolina at Chapel Hill,
Chapel Hill, NC 27599, USA
[4] Institute of Image Processing and Pattern Recognition,
Shanghai Jiao Tong University, Shanghai 200240, China

Abstract. Hippocampus segmentation from MR infant brain images is indispensable for studying early brain development. However, most of hippocampus segmentation methods were developed for adult brain images, which are not suitable for infant brain images of the first year due to low image contrast and variable structural patterns of early hippocampal development. To address these challenges, we propose a boundary regression method to detect hippocampal boundaries in the infant brain images, and then use the obtained boundaries to guide the deformable segmentation. The advantages of our segmentation method are: (1) different from the recently-developed atlas-based hippocampus segmentation methods, our method does not perform time-consuming deformable registrations; (2) different from the conventional point-regression-based boundary detection methods, our boundary regression method can predict the whole hippocampal boundary by a single regression model. Experiments on MR infant brain images from 2-week-old to 1-year-old show promising hippocampus segmentation results.

1 Introduction

In the first year of life, human brain undergoes a critical phase of postnatal brain development. To study brain development and detect neuro developmental disorders, identification of brain structures in MR images is a prerequisite. Among various structures, hippocampus plays an essential role in learning and memory functions of brain. Therefore, accurate hippocampus segmentation from infant brain images is highly desired for studying early brain development [1].

Currently, most of researches on hippocampus segmentation are based on atlases [2–4]. Due to the use of deformable registration between atlases and the target image, the atlas-based methods are often computationally-expensive. Besides, the existing methods are proposed mainly for hippocampus segmentation of the adult brain images. To date, it is still a challenging task to segment hippocampi in the infant brain images. The main

© Springer International Publishing Switzerland 2016
B. Menze et al. (Eds.): MCV Workshop 2015, LNCS 9601, pp. 146–154, 2016.
DOI: 10.1007/978-3-319-42016-5_14

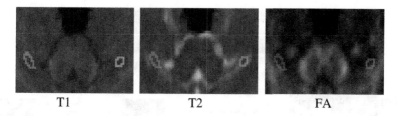

T1   T2   FA

Fig. 1. Illustration of hippocampi in T1, T2, and FA images of the same infant brain. The red and green contours indicate the left and right hippocampi, respectively. (Color figure online)

challenges include: (1) low image contrast, (2) ambiguous hippocampi boundary, and (3) small size of hippocampus with large nearby structures, as shown in Fig. 1.

To address the above challenges, inspired by [5], we propose a boundary regression method to vote the hippocampus boundaries of infant brain, and then use the obtained boundary voting map to guide a deformable model for final segmentation. Since the characteristics of the white matter, gray matter, and cerebral spinal fluid (CSF) change dynamically in the first year of life, we independently learn the boundary regression models and segment the hippocampi in different phases, i.e., (1) infantile phase (≤5 months), (2) isointense phase (6–8 months), and (3) early adult-like phase (≥9 months). Specifically, we first employ regression forests under an auto-context model to predict the hippocampus boundaries for each phase/age. In the implementation, we estimate a 3D displacement from any image voxel to the nearest hippocampus boundary point according to its local image appearance, and then cast a weighted vote on the predicted boundary point. In this way, we achieve a boundary voting map, which can enhance the hippocampus boundaries (as shown in Fig. 5(a)). We further adopt an auto-context model to incorporate the boundary prediction for refining the target boundary in the voting map. To take full advantage of T1, T2-weighted MR images, and fractional anisotropy (FA) image from diffusion tensor image of the same subject, we utilize all three modality images for boundary prediction. Then, guided by the refined boundary voting map, a deformable model is applied to obtain the final hippocampus segmentation. Note that, the boundary regression method in this paper will fuse the information of multi-modality images, instead of one-modality image [6]. In the experiments, our method achieved promising segmentation results for the infant brain images acquired from 2-week-old to 1-year-old.

2   Method

We aim to detect the hippocampus boundary by boundary regression with an auto-context model, and then segment the hippocampus on the boundary voting map by a deformable model. The proposed method consists of two components: (1) boundary regression with an auto-context model, and (2) deformable segmentation. Figure 2 shows the flowchart of our method.

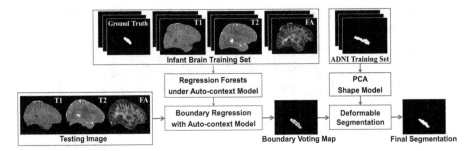

Fig. 2. The flowchart of our method. For simplicity, we only take the left hippocampus as an example.

2.1   Boundary Regression with Auto-Context Model

Local Boundary Regression: Regression forest is usually applied for point regression [7–9], which learns a non-linear mapping between local patches of image voxels and their respective displacements to a specific point. In this way, for 3D hippocampus boundary detection, these point regression methods need to train one regression forest for each of the massive boundary points (see examples of 2 boundary points in the left panel of Fig. 3), which makes these methods impractical due to the expensive computation. In this paper, we propose to train a regression forest to predict the 3D displacement from each image voxel to its nearest hippocampus boundary point by a local image patch (see the right panel of Fig. 3). Through a large number of votes at

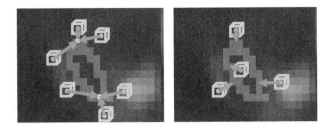

Fig. 3. Comparison of the conventional *point* regression (the left panel) and our *boundary* regression (the right panel). The red contour indicates the hippocampus boundary, and two white points in the left panel indicate two typical target boundary points. Each blue cube represents the image patch centered at an image voxel (i.e., the yellow point), and each green arrow represents the displacement vector from the patch center to a target boundary point. It is worth noting the difference between the two regression methods: the conventional *point* regression method targets for a specific boundary point, while our *boundary* regression method targets for the nearest boundary point from each patch center. (Color figure online)

predicted boundary points from different image voxels, our method can efficiently detect the whole hippocampus boundaries by a single regression forest.

In the training stage, to learn the regression forest, we randomly draw samples p_i ($i = 1, 2, \ldots, K$) near the manually-annotated hippocampus boundary using a Gaussian distribution for each training image. Mathematically, $p_i = q + N(q) \cdot \delta$, where q is a randomly-selected point on the manually-annotated hippocampus boundary, $N(q)$ is the normal direction of q regarding the manually-delineated target boundary, and $\delta = Gaussian\_rand(0, \sigma)$ is a random offset along the normal direction, determined by Gaussian distribution $\mathcal{N}(0, \sigma)$. Consequently, most samples are located around the target hippocampus boundary, which makes our regression model specific to hippocampus boundary detection. To represent each sample p_i, we extract randomly-generated, extended Haar feature vector F_i from a local image patch centered at p_i on the T1, T2, and FA modality images (i.e., $F_i = \left[F_{i,T1}^T F_{i,T2}^T F_{i,FA}^T \right]^T$). Note that, for each modality image, two types of randomly-generated, extended Haar features are achieved in the local image patch. The first type of extended Haar features consists of one block, which extracts the average image intensity within the block at the particular location. The second type of extended Haar features consists of two blocks, which extracts the difference of average intensity between the two blocks at two particular locations. To fully exploit the information within the local image patch, the polarity, center and size of each block are randomly sampled (as long as the block lies in the local patch). Also, we compute the displacement vector d_i from each sample p_i to the nearest hippocampus boundary point as the regression target. With all these Haar features and the corresponding 3D displacement vectors of all training samples, a regression forest R_0 (i.e., a set of decision trees) can be trained [10]. During this training stage, the regression forest only selects the useful features (adopted at the splitting node of each decision tree) from those randomly generated Haar features, and stores them tree-by-tree for the later testing stage.

In the testing stage, we use the testing image voxels in a region of interest (ROI) to predict the target hippocampus boundary. The ROI is a ring-shaped local region, centered at the initial shape of hippocampus. Here, the initial hippocampus shape is obtained by aligning a mean shape model onto the testing image according to the detected landmarks [11]. Since the initial shape is roughly near the target hippocampus boundary (i.e., with the DSC value between the initial shape and the manual segmentation as 0.60 for our dataset), the ROI can be considered around the hippocampus boundary. Note that the width of the ring-shaped ROI is 6 mm. Within the ROI, each image voxel $\hat{p}$ is employed to extract those useful Haar features $\hat{F}$ (previously recorded in the training stage) from its local patch. With the trained regression forest R_0, the extracted Haar feature vector $\hat{F}$ can be used to estimate the displacement from current image voxel to the potential nearest hippocampus boundary point, i.e., $\hat{d} = R_0(\hat{F})$. Since the points close to the target boundary can provide more information than those far-away points in boundary prediction, we adopt a weighted-voting strategy to vote for the target hippocampus boundary at the predicted position $\hat{p} + \hat{d}$. Here, the weight is inversely proportional to the Euclidean distance from $\hat{p}$ to the potential target boundary, and the weighted votes are accumulated on a 3D boundary voting map. By summing up all weighted votes from all voxels in the ROI of the testing image, we can finally get a boundary voting map for the hippocampi.

Refinement by Auto-Context Model: In the above boundary regression model, each image voxel independently predicts its target hippocampus boundary point, which tends to result in an incoherent boundary voting map (see Fig. 5(a)). To refine the hippocampus boundary in the voting map, we combine the boundary regression with the auto-context model [12], thus enforcing spatial constraint in the boundary regression to improve the regression result. The main idea is to sequentially train a set of regression forests $R_l(l = 0, 1, \ldots, L)$. The regression forest R_0 is trained only on the appearance features of the multi-modality images, as mentioned above. Each of other regression forests is trained with both the appearance features of the multimodality images and the context features of the intermediate displacement map estimated from the previous regression forest. The context features are computed as the randomly-generated, extended Haar features again. The flowchart of the auto-context model is shown in Fig. 4. Since the training of the auto-context model follows the same pipeline as the testing of the auto-context model, we just introduce the testing stage below.

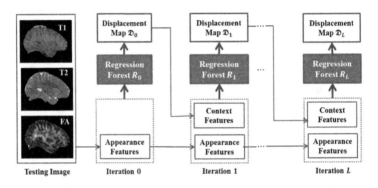

Fig. 4. The flowchart of the auto-context model in our proposed method.

In the testing stage, the learned regression forests are sequentially employed to estimate the 3D displacement vectors based on image voxels in the ring-shaped ROI. The generated displacement map is then used to extract context features. By combining these context features with the appearance features computed from the testing image, the next trained regression forest generates a new displacement map. By repeating this iterative step, a sequence of displacement maps can be generated.

Meanwhile, a sequence of refined boundary voting maps is also achieved with the estimated displacement vectors and the aforementioned weighted-voting strategy. The refined boundary voting maps under the auto-context model are illustrated in Fig. 5. The last boundary voting map includes the finally refined hippocampus boundary. In the experiment, we find that the training performance of our method converges by 3 iterations under the auto-context model. Therefore, we set the last iteration number L to 2.

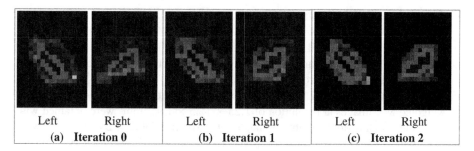

Left	Right	Left	Right	Left	Right
(a) Iteration 0		**(b) Iteration 1**		**(c) Iteration 2**	

Fig. 5. Boundary voting maps of one subject with auto-context model. The green curves represent the manually-delineated hippocampus boundaries. With the increase of iteration, the accuracy of the boundary voting map can be gradually improved. To hightlight the voted hippocampus boundaries, we only show the left and right hippocampus regions of the obtained boundary voting map at each iteration. (Color figure online)

2.2 Deformable Segmentation

The obtained boundary voting map highlights the target hippocampus boundary with high votes, which can be used as an external force to guide the active shape model (ASM) [13] for hippocampus segmentation.

Since the number of the infant subjects in our experiment is limited, i.e., 10 subjects. To establish the statistical shape model (shape priors) of hippocampus, we first build a PCA shape model based on hippocampus surfaces of 66 subjects from the ADNI dataset. Specifically, we extracted target hippocampus surfaces from 66 manually-segmented images by the marching cube algorithm [14]. One typical surface of these hippocampus surfaces is selected as a reference mesh and further smoothed. Here, the number of vertices on the reference mesh is 730. Then, a surface registration method is used to warp the reference mesh onto other hippocampus surface meshes for building surface correspondences. All these corresponded surfaces are affine aligned into a common space, and then used to build a PCA shape space with 98 % variation (with 6 modes).

In the testing stage, based on the initial shape inferred by the detected landmarks [11], each point of the hippocampus shape model can be independently deformed on the boundary voting map, by searching for a position with the maximal boundary votes along the respective surface normal direction. Then, the intermediate deformed shape is refined by the learned PCA shape model. By alternating the model deformation and the shape refinement, the deformation model can be iteratively driven towards the target hippocampus boundary, under the guidance from both the boundary voting map and the PCA shape space. The deformable segmentation converges until the intermediate deformed shape *no longer* changes. Besides the PCA shape analysis, others shape modeling methods, such as sparse shape composition [15], can also be used together with our boundary regression for deformable segmentation. Considering the efficiency and easiness, we use PCA in this paper.

3   Experimental Results

In the experiments, we use T1, T2 and FA images of 10 infant subjects at 2 weeks, 3 months, 6 months, 9 months and 12 months of age, respectively. T1- and T2-weighted images were both captured from a Siemens head-only 3T scanner. T1-weighted MR images at resolution of $1 \times 1 \times 1$ mm^3 were obtained with 144 sagittal slices, while T2-weighted MR images at resolution of $1.25 \times 1.25 \times 1.95$ mm^3 were obtained with 64 axis slices. Diffusion weighted images at resolution of $2 \times 2 \times 2$ mm^3 were obtained with 60 axial slices. Additionally, for each subject, T2-weighted MR images were aligned to the corresponding T1-weighted MR images; FA images were first aligned to the corresponding T2 images and then propagated to the corresponding T1 images. Since the T1, T2 and FA images from each subject shared the same brain anatomy, they can be accurately aligned with rigid registration by FLIRT [16] using mutual information as the similarity measure. All these images were isotropically resampled to $1 \times 1 \times 1$ mm^3. The image pre-processing steps (including skull stripping, bias-field correction, and histogram matching) were applied to each image. Besides, for each subject, the manual delineation of hippocampus is used as ground truth for evaluation.

We use leave-one-out cross-validations to evaluate our method. The parameter setting is as follows: the number of trees in each regression forest is 10; the maximum depth of each tree is 15; the number of candidate features for splitting node is 1000; the minimum number of samples in each leaf is 5; the patch size for extracting Haar features is 16 mm; the number of samples drawn from each training image is $K = 10000$; the number of iterations for auto-context model is 3; and the number of iterations for deformable model is 20.

To evaluate the respective roles of boundary regression and auto-context model, we apply the ASM model on **(1)** the original infant brain image, **(2)** boundary voting map without auto-context model, and **(3)** boundary voting map with 3-iteration auto-context model. (Considering different tissue contrasts of infant brain images at different ages, we take T2-weighted images as the original infant brain images for 2-week-old and 3-month-old, while T1-weighted images for 6-, 9-, and 12-month-old.) During the ASM-based deformable segmentation, in each original infant brain image, the deformable model searches for the maximal gradient along the normal direction of the surface model. By contrast, on the boundary voting map (with or without auto-context model), the deformable model searches for the maximal votes along the normal direction of the surface model. Note that, all methods adopt the same initial shape. As shown in Table 1, both the boundary regression and the auto-context model in our method are effective in improving the performance of hippocampus segmentation.

Our method is also quantitatively compared with the state-of-the-art multi-atlas based method for infant hippocampus segmentation, which uses sparse representation and deep learning for label propagation. From Table 2, we can see that our method achieves better performance on all 5 phases/ages.

Table 1. Comparison of two different components in our method in DSC (%).

Method	2-week	3-month	6-month	9-month	12-month
Original image + ASM	58.1 ± 10.2	60.8 ± 9.4	62.9 ± 7.3	65.7 ± 5.8	67.3 ± 5.2
Boundary regression + ASM	63.2 ± 7.1	66.7 ± 5.4	67.0 ± 5.2	70.6 ± 3.2	71.6 ± 2.9
Boundary regression + auto-context model + ASM	**68.5 ± 3.8**	**73.5 ± 1.3**	**74.8 ± 2.0**	**76.8 ± 1.2**	**76.9 ± 1.1**

Table 2. Comparison between our method and the state-of-the-art in DSC (%).

Method	2-week	3-month	6-month	9-month	12-month
Guo *et al.* [17]	62.3 ± 7.5	71.9 ± 1.5	71.8 ± 3.9	74.6 ± 2.9	*NA*
Our method	**68.5 ± 3.8**	**73.5 ± 1.3**	**74.8 ± 2.0**	**76.8 ± 1.2**	**76.9 ± 1.1**

4 Conclusions

In this paper, we present a new boundary regression method for hippocampus segmentation in MR infant brain images. Specifically, we learn a boundary regression model to predict the entire hippocampus boundary. Then, we integrate the regression model with the auto-context model to iteratively refine the boundary voting map. Finally, a deformable model is employed on the boundary voting map to achieve the final hippocampus segmentation. Validated on 10 subjects from 2-week-old to 1-year-old, our boundary regression based method achieves much better segmentation accuracy than the state-of-the-art method under comparison.

References

1. Thompson, D.K., Ahmadzai, Z.M., Wood, S.J., Inder, T.E., Warfield, S.K., Doyle, L.W., Egan, G.F.: Optimizing hippocampal segmentation in infants utilizing MRI post-acquisition processing. Neuroinformatics **10**, 173–180 (2012)
2. Coupé, P., Manjón, J.V., Fonov, V., Pruessner, J., Robles, M., Collins, D.: Nonlocal patch-based label fusion for hippocampus segmentation. In: Jiang, T., Navab, N., Pluim, J. P., Viergever, M.A. (eds.) MICCAI 2010, Part III. LNCS, vol. 6363, pp. 129–136. Springer, Heidelberg (2010)
3. Awate, S.P., Whitaker, R.T.: Multiatlas segmentation as nonparametric regression. IEEE Trans. Med. Imaging **33**(9), 1803–1817 (2014)
4. Wu, G., Wang, Q., Zhang, D., Nie, F., Huang, H., Shen, D.: A generative probability model of joint label fusion for multi-atlas based brain segmentation. Med. Image Anal. **18**, 881–890 (2014)
5. Criminisi, A., Shotton, J., Robertson, D., Konukoglu, E.: Regression forests for efficient anatomy detection and localization in CT studies. In: Menze, B., Langs, G., Tu, Z., Criminisi, A. (eds.) MICCAI 2010. LNCS, vol. 6533, pp. 106–117. Springer, Heidelberg (2011)

6. Shao, Y., Gao, Y., Yang, X., Shen, D.: CT prostate deformable segmentation by boundary regression. In: Menze, B., et al. (eds.) MCV 2014. LNCS, vol. 8848, pp. 127–136. Springer, Heidelberg (2014)

7. Chen, C., Xie, W., Franke, J., Grutzner, P., Nolte, L.-P., Zheng, G.: Automatic X-ray landmark detection and shape segmentation via data-driven joint estimation of image displacements. Med. Image Anal. **18**, 487–499 (2014)

8. Cootes, T.F., Ionita, M.C., Lindner, C., Sauer, P.: Robust and accurate shape model fitting using random forest regression voting. In: Fitzgibbon, A., Lazebnik, S., Perona, P., Sato, Y., Schmid, C. (eds.) ECCV 2012, Part VII. LNCS, vol. 7578, pp. 278–291. Springer, Heidelberg (2012)

9. Kohlberger, T., et al.: Automatic multi-organ segmentation using learning-based segmentation and level set optimization. In: Fichtinger, G., Martel, A., Peters, T. (eds.) MICCAI 2011, Part III. LNCS, vol. 6893, pp. 338–345. Springer, Heidelberg (2011)

10. Breiman, L.: Random forests. Mach. Learn. **45**, 5–32 (2001)

11. Gao, Y., Shen, D.: Context-aware anatomical landmark detection: application to deformable model initialization in prostate CT images. In: Wu, G., Zhang, D., Zhou, L. (eds.) MLMI 2014. LNCS, vol. 8679, pp. 165–173. Springer, Heidelberg (2014)

12. Tu, Z., Bai, X.: Auto-context and its application to high-level vision tasks and 3D brain image segmentation. IEEE Trans. Pattern Anal. Mach. Intell. **32**, 1744–1757 (2010)

13. Cootes, T.F., Taylor, C.J., Cooper, D.H., Graham, J.: Active shape models-their training and application. Comput. Vis. Image Underst. **61**, 38–59 (1995)

14. Lorensen, W.E., Cline, H.E.: Marching cubes: a high resolution 3D surface construction algorithm. SIGGRAPH Comput. Graph. **21**, 163–169 (1987)

15. Zhang, S., Zhan, Y., Dewan, M., Huang, J., Metaxas, D.N., Zhou, X.S.: Towards robust and effective shape modeling: sparse shape Compos. Med. Image Anal. **16**, 265–277 (2012)

16. Jenkinson, M., Bannister, P., Brady, M., Smith, S.: Improved optimization for the robust and accurate linear registration and motion correction of brain images. Neuroimage **17**, 825–841 (2002)

17. Guo, Y., Wu, G., Commander, L.A., Szary, S., Jewells, V., Lin, W., Shen, D.: Segmenting hippocampus from infant brains by sparse patch matching with deep-learned features. In: Golland, P., Hata, N., Barillot, C., Hornegger, J., Howe, R. (eds.) MICCAI 2014, Part II. LNCS, vol. 8674, pp. 308–315. Springer, Heidelberg (2014)

A Survey of Mathematical Structures for Extending 2D Neurogeometry to 3D Image Processing

Nina Miolane[1,2]([✉]) and Xavier Pennec[1]

[1] INRIA Asclepios, 2004 Route des Lucioles BP93, 06902 Sophia Antipolis, France
[2] Department of Statistics, Stanford University, Sequoia Hall, 390 Serra Mall,
Stanford, CA 94305-4065, USA
nina.miolane@inria.fr

Abstract. In the Big Data landscape, learning algorithms are often "black-boxes" and as such, hard to interpret. We need new constructive models, to eventually feed the Big Data framework. The emerging field of *Neurogeometry* provides inspiration for models in medical computer vision. Neurogeometry models the neuronal architecture of the visual cortex through Differential Geometry. First, Neurogeometry can explain visual phenomena like human perceptual completion. And second, it provides efficient algorithms for computer vision. Examples of applications are image completion (in-painting) and crossing-preserving smoothing. In *medical* computer vision, Neurogeometry is less known. One reason is that one often deals with 3D images, whereas Neurogeometry is essentially 2D (our retina is 2D). Moreover, the generalization to 3D is not mathematically straight-forward. This article presents the *theoretical framework of a 3D-Neurogeometry* inspired by the 2D case. The aim is to provide a *"theoretical toolbox"* and inspiration for new models in 3D medical computer vision.

1 Introduction

Machine learning algorithms using big data are often "black-boxes". Thus, they can be hard to interpret. There is still a need of constructive models, so that the big data framework can be fed by new structures. The visual cortex offers inspiration for new methods in (medical) computer vision. From the biological model of human vision, one builds a geometric model of the visual cortex. The geometric model is in turn implemented for computer vision purposes. This is the field of *(2D)-Neurogeometry*.

Biological Intuition Behind Neurogeometry. The geometric model of the visual cortex's is built as follows. From the biological point of view, neurons of the primary visual cortex $V1$ are local detectors called "point processors" [12]. They are retinotopically connected to small domains of the retina, called their "receptive field" [11]. Mathematically, this structure is an isomorphic map from

© Springer International Publishing Switzerland 2016
B. Menze et al. (Eds.): MCV Workshop 2015, LNCS 9601, pp. 155–167, 2016.
DOI: 10.1007/978-3-319-42016-5_15

the 2D retina to the 2D cortical layer. It means that each neuron is associated to a position in our retina $(x, y) \in \mathbb{R}^2$, or equivalently in our visual field.

Then, the neuron acts as a filter on the optical signal of the retina's photoreceptors. Its transfer function is called its "receptive profile". The so-called "simple neurons" of $V1$ have a highly anisotropic profile [11]. They are sensitive to the orientation $\theta \in S^1$ of the optical signal, in terms of the intensity gradient. A simple neuron is thus represented by the corresponding position $(x, y) \in \mathbb{R}^2$ of the retina and by the preferred orientation $\theta \in S^1$ of its filter [14].

Interestingly, Hubel and Wiesel have shown that neurons detecting all orientations at the same position (x, y) form an anatomical structure, called an "orientation hypercolumn" [10]. This discovery led to the Nobel Prize in 1981. It means that *the fiber bundle $\mathbb{R}^2 \times S^1$ is neurally implemented in the brain.*

Ultimately, one models the neuronal activity propagation in $\mathbb{R}^2 \times S^2$. The horizontal cortico-cortical connections of $V1$ are represented by a horizontal distribution in sub-Riemannian geometry [14]. The propagation of the cortical activity is then a propagation along sub-Riemannian geodesics [6].

Implementations of Neurogeometry for Computer Vision. One finds implementations of 2D-Neurogeometry in computer vision. For example, a sub-Riemannian diffusion process leads to algorithms for image completion or inpainting [3]. Fitting a sub-Riemannian geodesic enables contour completion [6]. Furthermore, a sub-Riemannian smoothing can smooth the image while preserving crossings [7]. But the framework lacks general applications in *medical* computer vision, although some exist [9]. One reason is that Neurogeometry is essentially 2D, as the retina is 2D. And the generalization of 2D-Neurogeometry to 3D-Neurogeometry is conceptually subtle. There is a need of a theoretical survey summarizing the mathematical structures in the 3D framework. The purpose of this paper is to fill this gap.

Contribution and Outline of the Paper. This paper aims to be a guide for understanding and generalizing 2D-Neurogeometry to 3D-Neurogeometry. It is a *theoretical toolbox of 3D-Neurogeometry* for: (1) conceiving new algorithms in medical computer vision; and (2) interpreting existing algorithms. In Sect. 2, we recall briefly some concepts of Differential Geometry. In Sect. 3, we describe 2D-Neurogeometry and its applications, as an introduction to the 3D case. In Sect. 4, we describe 3D-Neurogeometry and its possible applications.

2   Requirements of Differential Geometry

The following is summarized in Table 1 at the end of the section. We assume that the reader is familiar with the following concepts of Differential Geometry: manifolds, (principal) fiber bundles, (pseudo-) Riemannian manifolds [15], Lie groups, Lie algebra, bi-invariant (pseudo-)metrics [5,13], Lie group action on a manifold, homogeneous manifolds [1], sub-Riemannian manifolds [2]. Some are illustrated in Fig. 1.

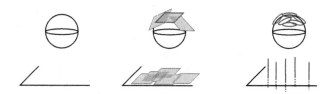

Fig. 1. Left: S^2 and $\mathbb{R}^2$ are manifolds. Center: tangent bundles of S^2 and $\mathbb{R}^2$. Right-top: principal bundle with base S^2 and structure group S^1. Right-bottom: principal bundle with base $\mathbb{R}^2$ and structure group $\mathbb{R}$. In all cases, the fibers are drawn in blue. (Color figure online)

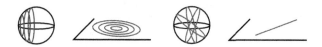

Fig. 2. From Left to Right. S^2 and $\mathbb{R}^2$ with action of $SO(2)$. The orbits are in blue and coincide with the curves created by the action of 1-parameter subgroups of $SO(2)$ (as $SO(2)$ is 1-dimensional). Riemannian geodesics on S^2 and $\mathbb{R}^2$ for standard induced metric from $\mathbb{R}^3$ on S^2 and the Euclidean metric on $\mathbb{R}^2$. (Color figure online)

The aforementioned structures are present simultaneously in the computational framework of Neurogeometry. They arise with their set of related curves, as shown in Table 1. Depending on the application for image processing, one is interested in computing one curve or another. Thus, on shall understand their differences and relations. Some curves are illustrated in Fig. 2.

3   The Example of 2D-Neurogeometry

This section serves as an introduction of the 3D case. An image processing pipeline using 2D-Neurogeometry usually follows three steps: 1. Lift (L), 2. Processing (P) and 3. Projection (P) (LPP-framework, see Fig. 3). These steps can be iterated [6,16] or not [4,7]. Biologically, the lift represents the activation of the neurons in V1. The processing of the lifted image represents the propagation of the neuronal activity in V1. The projection corresponds to our visual interpretation of the information given by the visual cortex after neuronal propagation.

First, we survey the mathematical structures (Subsects. 3.1, 3.2). We summarize them in Table 2. Then we present the LPP-frame of standard algorithms in 2D-Neurogeometry (Subsect. 3.3). Application-oriented readers can start with Subsect. 3.3, then go to Subsects. 3.1, 3.2.

3.1   Structures on the Lifted Space $SE(2) = \mathbb{R}^2 \times SO(2) = \mathbb{R}^2 \times S^1$

Group Actions. The law of $SE(2)$ is, for all $(t_1, R_1), (t_2, R_2) \in SE(2)$:

$$(t_1, R_1) * (t_2, R_2) = (R_1.t_2 + t_1, R_1.R_2)$$

Table 1. Curves related to the different structures of Differential Geometry in Neurogeometry. **For spaces:** M is a manifold, (P, M) a fiber bundle of base M, (M, G) is M endowed with a G action, (P, M, G) is a principal bundle of base M and structure group G, G is a Lie group. **For verticality/horizontality:** V^F, V^O, V and V^Δ: vertical in the sense of fibers, orbits, orbits=fibers (same notion for principal bundle), Δ-distribution. Same notations using H for horizontal. **For metric structures:** g^R is a (pseudo)-Riemannian metric, g^{SR} is a sub-Riemannian metric. **For curves:** γ denotes a notion of geodesics. We have γ^G, γ_e^G, γ^R, γ^{SR} for group geodesic, 1-parameter subgroup, Riemannian geodesics and sub-Riemannian geodesic.

	On M	On (P, M)	On (M, G)	On (P, M, G)	On G
No metric		• V^F-curves	• V^O-curves	• V-curves	• γ^G
			ex: γ^G-action	ex: γ^G-action	ex: γ_e^G
		• H^F-curves	• H^O-curves	• H-curves	
Metric g^R	• γ^R	• V^F-γ^R	• V^O-γ^R	• V-γ^R	IF g^R bi-inv.:
		• H^F-γ^R	• H^O-γ^R	• H-γ^R	$\gamma^G = \gamma^R$
SR-metric g^{SR}	• V^Δ-curves	IF $\Delta \perp$ fibers:	IF $\Delta \perp$ orbits:	IF $\Delta \perp$ fibers:	IF G Carnot:
	• H^Δ-curves	$V^\Delta = V^F$	$V^\Delta = V^O$	$V^\Delta = V$	$\exists\ g^{SR}$
	ex: γ^{SR}	$H^\Delta = H^F$	$H^\Delta = H^O$	$H^\Delta = H$	

In this law, we read the group actions on $SE(2)$ and their general properties. $SE(2)$ acts on itself through the left and right translations (freely and transitively). As a Lie subgroup, $SO(2)$ acts on $SE(2)$ on the left and right (freely but not transitively). Note that the right $SO(2)$-action is trivial on the $\mathbb{R}^2$ part. Moreover, the right $SO(2)$-action makes $SE(2)$ a principal bundle of base $\mathbb{R}^2$ and structure group $SO(2)$.

A Sub-Riemannian Metric and Two Riemannian Metrics. To introduce the sub-Riemannian metric, one first defines its horizontal distribution Δ. In 2D-Neurogeometry one takes the moving frame (X_1, X_2, X_3) on $\mathbb{R}^2 \times S^1$:

$$\begin{cases} X_1 = \cos\theta . \partial_x + \sin\theta . \partial_y, \\ X_2 = \partial_\theta, \\ X_3 = -\sin\theta . \partial_x + \cos\theta . \partial_y \end{cases}$$

to define $\Delta = (X_1, X_2)$. The sub-Riemannian metric g^{SR} is defined as the Euclidean metric on Δ. In the standard basis ∂_x, ∂_y, ∂_z, its inverse writes:

$$g^{SR}(x, y, \theta)^{ij} = \begin{pmatrix} \cos^2\theta & \sin\theta\cos\theta & 0 \\ \sin\theta\cos\theta & \sin^2\theta & 0 \\ 0 & 0 & 1 \end{pmatrix}$$

In practice, the sub-Riemannian metric is usually approximated the Riemannian metric g_ϵ^R whose inverse is [6]:

$$g_\epsilon^R(x, y, \theta)^{ij} = \begin{pmatrix} \cos^2\theta + \epsilon^2\sin^2\theta & (1-\epsilon^2)\sin\theta\cos\theta & 0 \\ (1-\epsilon^2)\sin\theta\cos\theta & \sin^2\theta + \epsilon^2\cos^2\theta & 0 \\ 0 & 0 & 1 \end{pmatrix}$$

In addition, one defines a left-invariant metric g_μ^R as:

$$g_\mu^R(0,0,0)_{ij} = \begin{pmatrix} \mu & 0 & 0 \\ 0 & \mu & 0 \\ 0 & 0 & 1 \end{pmatrix}$$

on the Lie algebra $\mathfrak{se}(2)$. Then, one propagates it on $SE(2)$ through left translations. g_μ^R is $(SE(2))$-left-invariant by construction. But g_μ^R is not $(SE(2))$-right-
invariant as there is no bi-invariant metric on $SE(2)$ [13]. g_μ^R is invariant by the
$SO(2)$-left and $SO(2)$-right actions.

A Survey of Curves. From Table 1 and the aforementioned structures, we survey the curves on $SE(2)$. We have group geodesics of $SE(2)$, Riemannian geodesics of g_μ^R, sub-Riemannian geodesics of g^{SR} and their Riemannian approximation
through g_ϵ^R. Group and Riemannian geodesics differ as g_μ^R is not bi-invariant.

w.r.t. the right $SO(2)$-action, some are vertical or horizontal (taken w.r.t. g_μ^R).
Examples of vertical group geodesics, vertical Riemannian geodesics for g_μ^R and
vertical sub-Riemannian geodesics for g^{SR} are orbits of the $SO(2)$-action. Examples of horizontal group geodesics, horizontal Riemannian geodesics for g_μ^R are
straight lines between two translations. Examples of horizontal sub-Riemannian
geodesics for g^{SR} are integral curves of X_1.

w.r.t. Δ, some are Δ-vertical or Δ-horizontal. There is no Δ-vertical group
geodesics, and no Δ-vertical Riemannian geodesic. Example of Δ-horizontal
group geodesics and Δ-horizontal Riemannian geodesic for g_μ^R are orbits of the
right $SO(2)$-action. Sub-Riemannian geodesics are always Δ-horizontal.

3.2 Structures on the Image Domain $\mathbb{R}^2$

Projecting $\mathbb{R}^2 \times S^1$ along the fibers S^1 gives $\mathbb{R}^2$. Equivalently, we can quotient
$SE(2)$ by the $SO(2)$-right. The residual left $SE(2)$-action on $\mathbb{R}^2$ is: $(t, R) \circ x =
R.x + t$. We read the related left $SO(2)$-action. Regarding the metric structures,
g_μ^R was right $SO(2)$-invariant. Thus the projection is a Riemannian submersion
for g_μ^R. It induces a Riemannian metric on $\mathbb{R}^2$ which is the Euclidean metric.
Projecting the horizontal Riemannian geodesics gives linear curves in $\mathbb{R}^2$. The
projection of the sub-Riemannian geodesics gives the elastica curves [6], which
can be linear or curvilinear.

3.3 The Three Steps: LPP Framework for 2D

First Step: Lift (L). The image domain $D \subset \mathbb{R}^2$ is lifted to $\tilde{D} \in \mathbb{R}^2 \times S^1$ [6]
(positions and orientations taken with directions). The lift is implemented by
detecting the direction of the intensity gradient:

$$\frac{\nabla I}{||\nabla I||} = (-\sin\theta, \cos\theta)$$

Table 2. Structures of 2D-Neurogeometry. Use Table 1 to get the related curves.

	Actions	Metrics
$SE(2) = \mathbb{R}^2 \times S^1$	• left, right translations of $SE(2)$	• g_μ^R
	• left, right actions of $SO(2)$	• g^{SR}
		• g_ϵ^{SR}
$\mathbb{R}^2$	• left action of $SE(2)$	• Euclidean metric (projection of g_μ^R)
	• left action of $SO(2)$	

at each point $(x, y) \in D$. Then D is mapped to a surface $\tilde{D}$: $(x, y) \mapsto (x, y, \theta(x, y))$ in $\mathbb{R}^2 \times S^1$. At the end of this step, the intensity is a function of $\tilde{D}$.

Alternatively, one can lift to the projective tangent bundle $PT\mathbb{R}^2 = SE(2)/\mathbb{Z}_2$ (positions and orientations taken without directions)[4]. Whether one should use $SE(2)$ of $PT\mathbb{R}^2$ is discussed here [4](Remark 4, 13).

Second Step: Processing (P). First, the processing can be the evolution of partial differential equations (PDEs) with sub-Riemannian operators. For example, the sub-Riemannian diffusion is defined with the sub-Riemannian Laplacian $\Delta_{SR} = X_1^2 + X_2^2$. Depending on the goal of the processing, one adds drift (also called convection) to the PDE: there is drift for completion purposes [4] and for enhancement [9]. Equivalently, one can formulate this step as an oriented random walk. One writes the corresponding Kolmogorov equations.

Some PDEs are computed with the lifted intensity $I(x, y, \theta)$. In-painting methods provide examples: one "paints" directly in the lifted space [4]. Others compute with the activity function: $u(x, y, \theta) = u(x, y, \theta)\delta_\Sigma$ where $u(x, y, \theta) = |X_3(\theta).\nabla I(x, y)|$. In-painting methods provide also examples of this approach [16]. The corrupted image has a hole in $\tilde{D}$. The activity propagation amounts to "fill the hole" by a minimal surface. Then, one "paints" the surface by linking the isolevel sets with sub-Riemannian geodesics.

Then, the processing can be curve fitting. Which curve do we fit? One can fit a sub-Riemannian geodesic, as in the second example of in-painting above [16]. Another example is contour completion [6]. One can also fit a Riemannian geodesic or a group geodesic for enhancement of 1-dimensional structures. A comparison of the two suggests that one should prefer the group geodesic [8,9](called the "exponential curve" here).

Third Step: Projection (P). The processed lifted image on $\mathbb{R}^2 \times S^1$ is projected to a "standard" image defined on $\mathbb{R}^2$. The projection can be done in two different ways. First, one can use the "verticality" along fibers of the bundle $\mathbb{R}^2 \times S^1$. In this case, one projects along the fiber S^1, choosing a θ that maximizes a likelihood criterion [3]. Second, one can use the "Δ-verticality" of sub-Riemannian geometry. In this case, one projects along the normal of the

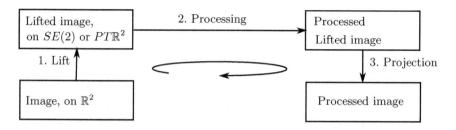

Fig. 3. The 3 steps of image processing in 2D-Neurogeometry: LPP framework.

horizontal distribution Δ through a concentration scheme [16]. This allows for several maxima at each point, i.e. crossings on the image.

4   A Theoretical Toolbox for 3D-Neurogeometry

As implemented by now [7,9], image processing pipelines using 3D-neurogeometry also follows the three same steps: 1. Lift (L), 2. Processing (P) and 3. Projection (P) (see Fig. 4). This steps could be iterated or not. The difference with the 2D-neurogeometry however is the Processing. In this step, there is an additional level of structure in 3D-Neurogeometry w.r.t. the 2D case.

As in the 2D-case, we first survey the mathematical structures and summarize them in Table 5 (Subsects. 4.1, 4.2, 4.3). Then we present the LPP-frame of a 3D-Neurogeometry (Subsect. 4.4). Application-oriented readers can read Subsect. 4.4 first, and then go to Subsects. 4.1, 4.2, 4.3.

4.1   Structures on the Lie Group $SE(3) = \mathbb{R}^3 \times SO(3)$

Group Actions. The law of $SE(3)$ is, for all $(t_1, R_1), (t_2, R_2) \in \mathbb{R}^3 \times SO(3)$:

$$(t_1, R_1) * (t_2, R_2) = (R_1.t_2 + t_1, R_1.R_2).$$

We read the group actions on $SE(3)$ and their properties (see Table 3).

As a Lie group, $SE(3)$ acts on itself through left and right translations. As subgroups of $SE(3)$, $SO(3)$ and $SO(2)$ also act on $SE(3)$, on the left and right. The right $SO(3)$-action makes $SE(3)$ a trivial principal bundle over $\mathbb{R}^3$ with structure group $SO(3)$. The right $SO(2)$-action on $SE(3)$ makes the $SE(3)$ a principal bundle over $\mathbb{R}^3 \times S^2$ with structure group $SO(2)$.

A Left-Invariant Metric and a Bi-Invariant Pseudo-Metric. As in the 2D case, one defines the left-invariant metric g_μ^R on $SE(3)$. g_μ^R is left-invariant by construction. But g_μ^R is not right-invariant.

g_μ^R is invariant by the left and right $SO(3)$-actions. The left $SO(3)$-invariance comes from the left invariance of g_μ^R. The right $SO(3)$-invariance is shown considering the right action on the parts $\mathbb{R}^3$ and $SO(3)$ separately, as g_μ^R is diagonal. Consequently, g_μ^R is also invariant by left and right $SO(2)$-actions.

Table 3. Properties of group actions on $SE(3)$. "Isotropy" means the isotropy groups. Actions on the $\mathbb{R}^3$-part of $SE(3) = \mathbb{R}^3 \times SO(3)$ are the main distinction between Left and Right. "Fundamental" denotes the fundamental representation on $\mathbb{R}^3$, and "Trivial" the trivial representation on $\mathbb{R}^3$.

		Free	Transitive	Orbits	Isotropy	Quotient	On $\mathbb{R}^3$-part
$SE(3)$-actions	**Left**	yes	yes	$SE(3)$	$\{e\}$	$\{[e]\}$	fundamental
	Right	yes	yes	$SE(3)$	$\{e\}$	$\{[e]\}$	trivial
$SO(3)$-actions	**Left**	yes	no	$\sim SO(3)$	$\{e\}$	$\mathbb{R}^3$	fundamental
	Right	yes	no	$\sim SO(3)$	$\{e\}$	$\mathbb{R}^3$	trivial
$SO(2)$-actions	**Left**	yes	no	$\sim SO(2)$	$\{e\}$	$\mathbb{R}^3 \times S^2$	fundamental
	Right	yes	no	$\sim SO(2)$	$\{e\}$	$\mathbb{R}^3 \times S^2$	trivial

As opposed as the $2D$ case, there exist bi-invariant pseudo-metrics on $SE(3)$. We refer to [13] for their explicit construction. A possible choice is:

$$g^{BI}(0, \mathbb{I}_3)_{ij} = \begin{pmatrix} 0 & \mathbb{I}_3 \\ \mathbb{I}_3 & 0 \end{pmatrix}$$

known as the Klein form. Here $\mathbb{I}_3$ is the 3D identity matrix.

A Survey of Curves on $SE(3)$. From Table 1 and the aforementioned structures, we survey the curves on $SE(3)$. We have the group geodesics of $SE(3)$, the Riemannian geodesics of g_μ^R an the pseudo-Riemannian geodesics of g^{BI}. The group geodesics coincide with the pseudo-Riemannian ones, but differ from the Riemannian ones [15] (see Table 1).

w.r.t. a $SO(3)$- or $SO(2)$-action, some of these curves are vertical, some are horizontal (taken w.r.t. g_μ^R). Examples of vertical group geodesics are the orbits of the $SO(2)$-action or the action of the group geodesics of $SO(3)$. Examples of horizontal group geodesics are those generated by an element of the Lie algebra of the translations.

4.2   Structures on the Lifted Space $\mathbb{R}^3 \times S^2$ and on $\mathbb{R}^3$

We go from $SE(3)$ to $\mathbb{R}^3 \times S^2$, by quotienting the right $SO(2)$-action. The quotient is implemented by choosing an origin in $\mathbb{R}^3 \times S^2$, usually $(0, a)$. An element $(x, n) \in \mathbb{R}^3 \times S^2$ is represented as the result of the action of the corresponding (x, R) on $(0, a)$, where R is precisely the rotation bringing a onto n.

Induced Group Actions. The induced action of $SE(3)$ on $\mathbb{R}^3 \times S^2$ writes, for all $(t, R) \in SE(3)$ and $(x, n) \in \mathbb{R}^3 \times S^2$:

$$(t, R) * (x, n) = (R.x + t, R.n)$$

We read the group actions on $\mathbb{R}^3 \times S^2$ and their properties (see Table 4).

The $SE(3)$-action is transitive on $\mathbb{R}^3 \times S^2$. It makes $\mathbb{R}^3 \times S^2$ a homogeneous space. As the isotropy group is $SO(2)$ everywhere, the orbit-stabilizer theorem gives: $\mathbb{R}^3 \times S^2 = SE(3)/SO(2)$. Moreover, it provides the justification of the choice of an origin $(0, a)$ in computer vision algorithms. All points are equivalent in a homogeneous space. Computations do not depend on the choice of origin.

Table 4. Induced group actions on $\mathbb{R}^3 \times S^2$. Note that there are no more right actions, as $SO(2)$ is not a normal group of $SO(3)$ nor $SE(3)$. "Isotropy" means the "isotropy groups". "Fundamental" denotes the fundamental representation on $\mathbb{R}^3$.

		Free	Trans.	Orbits	Isotropy	Quotient	On $\mathbb{R}^3$-part
$SE(3)$-**action**	**Left**	no	yes	$\mathbb{R}^3 \times S^2$	$SO(2)$	$\{[e]\}$	fundamental
$SO(3)$-**action**	**Left**	no	no	$\sim SO(3)/SO(2)$	$SO(2)$	$\mathbb{R}^3$	fundamental

Induced Riemannian and Pseudo-Riemannian Metrics. g_μ^R was invariant by the right $SO(2)$-action. Thus, the projection onto $\mathbb{R}^3 \times S^2$ is a Riemannian submersion for g_μ^R. It induces a Riemannian metric on $\mathbb{R}^3 \times S^2$, still denoted g_μ^R. g_μ^R is still $SE(3)$- and $SO(3)$- invariant.

Similarly, g^{BI} was invariant by the right $SO(2)$-action. It induces a Riemannian pseudo-metric on $\mathbb{R}^3 \times S^2$, which is still $SE(3)$- and $SO(3)$- invariant.

A Sub-Riemannian Metric. As in 2D, one defines a sub-Riemannian metric g^{SR} on $\mathbb{R}^3 \times S^2$ by first defining Δ. We take $(X_1, X_2, X_3, X_4, X_5)$ on $\mathbb{R}^3 \times S^2$ as:

$$
\begin{cases}
X_1 = \cos\theta\cos\phi.\partial_x + \cos\theta\sin\phi.\partial_y - \sin\theta.\partial_z, \\
X_2 = -\sin\phi.\partial_x + \cos\phi.\partial_y, \\
X_3 = \partial_\theta, \\
X_4 = \partial_\phi, \\
X_5 = \sin\theta\cos\phi.\partial_x + \sin\theta\sin\phi.\partial_y + \cos\theta.\partial_z
\end{cases}
$$

and $\Delta = \mathrm{Span}\{X_1, X_2, X_3, X_4\}$. g^{SR} is defined as the Euclidean metric on Δ. As in the 2D-case, it would be approximated by a Riemannian metric in practice.

A Survey of Curves. From Table 1 and the aforementioned structures, we survey the curves on $SE(3)$. However, we have a new class of curves in 3D-Neurogeometry w.r.t. 2D-Neurogeometry: the curves of the lifted space $\mathbb{R}^3 \times S^2$ that are projection of curves of $SE(3)$, as the projection of the group geodesics.

In the following, "verticality" and "horizontality" are taken w.r.t. the right $SO(2)$-action. Projecting horizontal (g_μ^R) Riemannian geodesics gives *generalized*

Riemannian geodesics. Projecting horizontal (for g^{BI}) pseudo-Riemannian geodesics gives *generalized pseudo-Riemannian geodesics*. More precisely, a smooth horizontal curve in $SE(3)$ is a (pseudo-) Riemannian geodesics if and only if it is a (pseudo-) Riemannian geodesics in $\mathbb{R}^3 \times S^2$. The projection of vertical curves are points. The projection of a curve that is vertical at one point has a "cusp".

Ultimately, we have the curves that are Δ-horizontal in the sense of the sub-Riemannian geometry. Among them, we have sub-Riemannian geodesics.

4.3   Structures on the Image Domain $\mathbb{R}^3$

The previous structures are projected to $\mathbb{R}^3$, using the projection of the trivial bundle $\mathbb{R}^3 \times S^2$ on the first component. In particular, projecting the previous curves give curves in $\mathbb{R}^3$. We have: the projection of the sub-Riemannian geodesics (an equivalent of 2D elastica curves), the double-projection of the group geodesics (equivalently the double-projection of the pseudo-Riemannian curves for g^{BI}), the double-projection of the Riemannian geodesics for g_μ^R.

Table 5. Structures of 3D-Neurogeometry. Use Table 1 to get the related curves.

	Actions	Metrics
$SE(3)$	• left, right translations of $SE(3)$	• g_μ^R
	• left, right actions of $SO(3)$	• g^{BI}
	• left, right actions of $SO(2)$	
$\mathbb{R}^3 \times S^2$	• left action of $SE(3)$	• projection of g_μ^R
	• left action of $SO(3)$	• projection of g^{BI}
		• g^{SR}
		• g_ϵ^{SR}
$\mathbb{R}^3$	• left action of $SE(3)$	• Euclidean metric
	• left action of $SO(3)$	(double-projection of g_μ^R)

4.4   The Three Steps: LPP Framework for 3D

First Step: Lift (L). As in 2D, one lifts the medical image defined on $D \subset \mathbb{R}^3$ to an image defined on $\tilde{D} \subset \mathbb{R}^3 \times S^2$, using the gradient direction at each $(x, y, z) \in D$:

$$\frac{\nabla I}{||\nabla I||} = (\sin \theta \cos \phi, \sin \theta \sin \phi, \cos \theta)$$

Second Step: Processing (P). First, as in 2D, the processing could be performed on $\mathbb{R}^3 \times S^2$ without taking into account the $SE(3)$ structure. One would only consider the sub-Riemannian structure on the lifted space $\mathbb{R}^3 \times S^2$. In doing so, one could define sub-Riemannian partial differential equations as in 2D-Neurogeometry, using the X_i as differential operators. For in-painting purposes, the 2D work of [3,16] provides intuition. Similarly, one could add drift (or convection) depending on the application.

Then, in contrast to 2D, the processing *can* be performed on $SE(3)$. This is done by embedding $\mathbb{R}^3 \times S^2$ in $SE(3)$ as the quotient of $SE(3)$ by a $SO(2)$-action. Then, performing $SO(2)$-invariant computations on $SE(3)$ is equivalent to performing computations on $\mathbb{R}^3 \times S^2$. The advantage is that one has more structures, e.g. more curves for curve fitting (compare Subsects. 2.2 and 3.4).

This is the first main distinction between the 2D and the 3D case. In 2D-Neurogeometry, we have one (trivial) quotient of $\mathbb{R}^2 \times S^2$. In contrast in 3D-Neurogeometry, one has two successive quotients of $SE(3) = \mathbb{R}^3 \times SO(3)$.

The second distinction is the existence of bi-invariant pseudo-metrics g^{BI} in the 3D-case, but not in the 2D-case [13]. As such, g^{BI} could represent a new powerful tool of 3D-Neurogeometry. We note that in medical computer vision, the bi-invariant pseudo-metric g^{BI} is rarely used as opposed to algorithms in robotics [17]. Considering its bi-invariance property, it would be interesting to consider it for the computations. For example, g^{BI} characterizes the group geodesics of $SE(3)$: this could simplify computations. g^{BI} could replace the use of g_μ^R as an auxiliary metric, suppressing the need of a choice of μ.

Third Step: Projection (P). The projection of the lifted image to an image defined on $\mathbb{R}^3$ could be defined in two different ways, exactly as in the 2D-case.

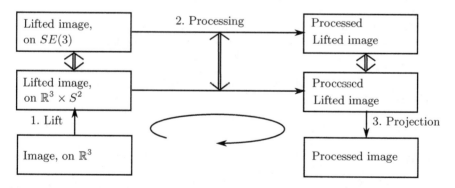

Fig. 4. The 3 steps of image processing for 3D-Neurogeometry: LPP framework.

5   Conclusion

This paper is a *theoretical toolbox* for creating new algorithms in 3D medical computer vision. We have described the mathematical structures arising in the generalization of (2D-)Neurogeometry to 3D images.

References

1. Alekseevsky, D., Kriegl, A., Losik, M., Michor, P.W.: The Riemannian geometry of orbit spaces: metric, geodesics, and integrable systems. Publicationes Mathematicae Debrecen **62**(3-4), 1–30 (2003)
2. Bellaïche, A., Risler, J.J.: Sub-Riemannian Geometry. Progress in Mathematics, vol. 144. Birkhäuser (1996)
3. Boscain, U., Chertovskih, R.A., Gauthier, J.P., Remizov, A.O.: Hypoelliptic diffusion and human vision: a semidiscrete new twist. J. Imaging Sci. Soc. Ind. Appl. Math. **7**(2), 669–695 (2014)
4. Boscain, U.V., Duplaix, J., Gauthier, J.P., Rossi, F.: Anthropomorphic image reconstruction via hypoelliptic diffusion. SIAM J. Control Optim. **50**(3), 1309–1336 (2012)
5. Bourbaki, N.: Lie Groups and Lie Algebras: Chap. 1–3. Hermann, Elements of mathematics (1989)
6. Citti, G., Sarti, A.: A cortical based model of perceptual completion in the roto-translation space. J. Math. Imaging Vis. **24**(3), 307–326 (2006)
7. Duits, R., Franken, E.: Left-invariant parabolic evolutions on se (2) and contour enhancement via invertible orientation scores. Part I: Linear left-invariant diffusion equations on se(2). Q. Appl. Math. **68**, 255–292 (2010)
8. Duits, R., Franken, E.: Left-invariant parabolic evolutions on se(2) and contour enhancement via invertible orientation scores. Part II : non linear left invariant diffusion equations on invertible orientation scores. Q. Appl. Math. **68**, 293–331 (2010)
9. Duits, R., Franken, E.: Left-invariant diffusions on the space of positions and orientations and their application to crossing-preserving smoothing of HARDI images. Int. J. Comput. Vis. **92**(3), 231–264 (2011)
10. Hubel, D., Willmer, C., Rutter, J.: Orientation columns in macaque monkey visual cortex demonstrated by the 2-deoxyglucose autoradiographic technique. Nature **269**, 22 (1977)
11. Jones, J.P., Palmer, L.A.: An evaluation of the two-dimensional Gabor filter model of simple receptive fields in cat striate cortex. J. Neurophysiol. **58**(6), 1233–1258 (1987)
12. Koenderink, J., van Doorn, A.: Representation of local geometry in the visual system. Biol. Cybern. **55**(6), 367–375 (1987)
13. Miolane, N., Pennec, X.: Computing bi-invariant pseudo-metrics on lie groups for consistent statistics. Entropy J. Multi. Digital Publishing Inst. **17**(4), 1850–1881 (2015)
14. Petitot, J.: Neurogeometry of neural functional architectures. Chaos, Solitons Fractals **50**, 75–92 (2013)
15. Postnikov, M.: Geometry VI: Riemannian Geometry. Encyclopaedia of Mathematical Sciences. Springer, Heidelberg (2001)

16. Sanguinetti, G., Citti, G., Sarti, A.: Image completion using a diffusion driven mean curvature flowing a sub-Riemannian space. In: Proceedings of the International Conference on Computer Vision Theory and Applications, VISApp. 2008, Funchal, vol. 2, pp. 46–53 (2008)
17. Zefran, M., Kumar, V., Crocke, C.: On the generation of smooth tridimensional rigid body motions. IEEE Trans. Robot. Autom. **14**(4), 576–589 (1995)

Efficient 4D Non-local Tensor Total-Variation for Low-Dose CT Perfusion Deconvolution

Ruogu Fang[1]([✉]), Ming Ni[2], Junzhou Huang[3], Qianmu Li[2], and Tao Li[1]

[1] School of Computing and Information Sciences,
Florida International University, Miami, USA
rfang@cs.fiu.edu
[2] School of Computer Science and Engineering,
Nanjing University of Science and Technology, Nanjing, China
[3] Department of Computer Science and Engineering,
University of Texas at Arlington, Arlington, USA

Abstract. Tensor total variation deconvolution has been recently proposed as a robust framework to accurately estimate the hemodynamic parameters in low-dose CT perfusion by fusing the local anatomical structure correlation and the temporal blood flow continuation. However the locality property in the current framework constrains the search for anatomical structure similarities to the local neighborhood, missing the global and long-range correlations in the whole anatomical structure. This limitation has led to the noticeable absence or artifacts of delicate structures, including the critical indicators for the clinical diagnosis of cerebrovascular diseases. In this paper, we propose an extension of the TTV framework by introducing 4D non-local tensor total variation into the deconvolution to bridge the gap between non-adjacent regions of the same tissue classes. The non-local regularization using tensor total variation term is imposed on the spatio-temporal flow-scaled residue functions. An efficient algorithm and the implementation of the non-local tensor total variation (NL-TTV) reduce the time complexity with the fast similarity computation, the accelerated optimization and parallel operations. Extensive evaluations on the clinical data with cerebrovascular diseases and normal subjects demonstrate the importance of non-local linkage and long-range connections for the low-dose CT perfusion deconvolution.

1 Introduction

Stroke and cerebrovascular diseases are the leading causes of serious, long-term disability in the United States, with an average occurrence in the population at every 40 s. In the world, 15 million people suffer from stroke each year and among these, 5 million die and another 5 million are permanently disabled. The mantra in stroke care is "time is brain". With each passing minute, more brain cells are irretrievably lost and, therefore, timely diagnosis and treatment are essential to increase the chances for recovery. As a critical step in the stroke care, imaging of the brain provides important quantitative measurements for the physicians to

© Springer International Publishing Switzerland 2016
B. Menze et al. (Eds.): MCV Workshop 2015, LNCS 9601, pp. 168–179, 2016.
DOI: 10.1007/978-3-319-42016-5_16

"see" what is occurring in the brain. Computed tomography perfusion (CTP), with its rapid imaging speed, high resolution and wide availability, has been one of the most widely available and most frequently used imaging modality for stroke care.

Unfortunately, the associated high radiation exposure in CTP have caused adverse biological effects such as hair loss, skin burn, and more seriously, increased cancer risk. Lowering the radiation exposure would reduce the potential health hazard to which the patients are exposed, improve healthcare quality and safety, as well as make CTP modality fully utilized for a wider population. However, low radiation dose in CTP will inevitably lead to noisy and less accurate quantifications. There are various efforts to reduce the necessary radiation dose in CTP, mostly in two classes; noise reduction at the reconstruction stage [1–5], and stabilization at the deconvolution stage [6–9].

While the first class of approaches does not solve the inherent instability problem in the quantification (deconvolution) process of CTP, the second class of approaches directly addresses this instability issue. Among these methods, the information redundancy and sparsity is a property that has shed light into the low-dose quantification problems [7,8,10,11], but the sparsity frameworks needs training data for dictionary learning. In another line of work, tensor total variation (TTV) deconvolution [9,12] has been recently pro posed to significantly reduce the radiation dosage in CTP with improved robustness and quantitative accuracy by integrating the anatomical structure correlation and the temporal blood flow model. The anatomical structure of the brain encompasses long-range similarity of the same tissue classes, as shown in Fig. 1(a). However the locality property of the current TTV algorithm limits the search for similar patterns in the 4-connected adjacent neighborhood, neglecting the long-range or global correlations of the entire brain structure. This locality limitation has led to noticeable absence or artifact of the delicate structures, such as the capillary, the insula and the parietal lobe, which are critical indicators for the clinical diagnosis of cerebrovascular diseases. Figure 1(b) shows the importance of accurate depiction of hemodynamic parameters. The delicate vascular and cerebral structures are critical biomarkers of the existence and severity of the cerebrovascular diseases. Naturally, integrating the long-range and non-local correlation into the estimation process of the hemodynamic parameters would yield more precise depiction of the pathological regions in the brain.

In this paper, we propose a fast non-local tensor total variation (NL-TTV) deconvolution method to improve the clinical value of low-dose CTP. Instead of restricting the regularization of residue functions to the adjoining voxels in the spatial domain and neighboring frames in the temporal domain, the long-range dependency and the global connections in the spatial and temporal dimensions are both considered. While non-local total variation and TTV are not new concepts, the integration of the two methods in a spatio-temporal framework to regularize the flow-scaled residue impulse functions has never been proposed, and can make significant improvement in the perfusion parameter estimation.

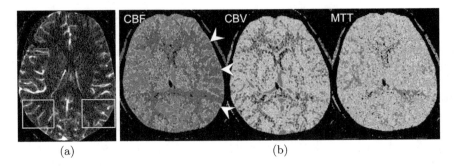

Fig. 1. (a) The illustration of long-range similarity in the brain. The red and yellow boxes show the non-local regions which have similar patterns. (b) Perfusion parameter maps (CBF - cerebral blood flow, CBV - cerebral blood volume, and MTT - mean transit time) of a 22-year old with severe left middle cerebral artery (MCA) stenosis. Arrows indicate the regions with ischemia. The shape, intensity and coverage of the capillary and vessels are evidence of ischemia in the left hemisphere (right side of the image). (Color figure online)

Furthermore, the efficient algorithm to accelerate the non-local TTV would make the proposed algorithm clinical valuable.

The contribution of this work is two-fold: First, the long-range and global connections are explored to leverage the anatomical symmetry and structural similarity of the same tissue classes in both the spatial and the temporal dimensions. Second, efficient parallel implementation and similarity computation using window offsets reduce the time complexity of the non-local algorithm. The extensive experiments on low-dose CTP clinical data of subjects with cerebrovascular diseases and normal subjects are performed. The experiments demonstrate the superiority of the non-local framework, compared with the local TTV method. The advantages include more accurate preservation of the fine structures and higher spatial resolution for the low-dose data.

2   Efficient Non-local Tensor Total Variation Deconvolution

In this section, we will first briefly review the tensor total variation model for the low-dose CTP and discuss its deficiency in accurate estimation of delicate structure and distinguishing pattern complexities. Based on that, we will introduce the proposed efficient non-local tensor total variation model, followed by experimental results, discussion and conclusion.

2.1   Tensor Total Variation Deconvolution

To reduce the radiation dose in CT perfusion imaging, Tensor total variation (TTV) [9] is recently proposed to efficiently and robustly estimate the hemodynamic parameters. It integrates the anatomical structure correlation and the temporal continuation of the blood flow signal. The TTV algorithm optimizes a cost function with one linear system for the deconvolution and one smoothness regularization term, as below:

$$K_{TTV} = \underset{K \in \mathbb{R}^{T \times N}}{\arg \min}(\frac{1}{2}\|AK - C\|_2^2 + \|K\|_{TTV}^{\gamma}) \tag{1}$$

The first term is the temporal convolution model. In this term, $A \in \mathbb{R}^{T \times T}$ is a block-circulant matrix representing the arterial input function (AIF), which is the input signal to the linear time-invariant system of the capillary bed. The block-circulant format makes the deconvolution insensitive to delays in the AIF. $C \in \mathbb{R}^{T \times N}$ is the contrast agent concentration (CAC) curves of all the voxels in the volume of interest (VOI). Both A and C are extracted from the CTP data. $K \in \mathbb{R}^{T \times N}$ is the unknown of this optimization problem - the flow-scaled residue functions of the VOI. Here T is the duration of the signal, and $N = N_1 \times N_2 \times N_3$ is the total number of voxels in the sagittal, coronal and axial directions.

The second term is the tensor total variation regularizer. The TTV regularization is defined as

$$\|K\|_{TTV}^{\gamma} = \sum_{i,j,k,t} \sqrt{\sum_{d=1}^{4}(\gamma_d \nabla_d \tilde{K}_{i,j,k,t})^2} \tag{2}$$

with ∇_d is the forward finite difference operator in the dth dimension, and $\tilde{K} \in \mathbb{R}^{T \times N_1 \times N_2 \times N_3}$ is the 4-dimensional volume reshaped from matrix K with temporal signal for one dimension and spatial signal for three dimensions. t, i, j, k are the indices for the temporal and spatial dimensions. The outside summation means that the square root of the sum of the first order derivative is summed over all the temporal points t and spatial voxels i, j, k of $\tilde{K}$. L_1 norm is used in the forward finite difference operator ∇_d to preserve the edges, and the regularization parameters γ_d designates the regularization strength for each dimension. Cerebral blood flow (CBF) maps can be computed from K as the maximum value at each voxel over time. More details about the TTV framework can be found in [9].

While TTV achieves significant performance improvement on the digital brain phantom and low- and ultra-low dose clinical CTP data at 30, 15 and 10 mAs [9], the locality property of the tensor total variation regularization limits the capability of preserving the small and fine anatomical structures, details and texture in the brain, including the capillary, the insula and the parietal lobe, which are essential indicators of the location and severity of the ischemic or hemorrhagic stroke. It may also create new distortions, such as blurring, staircase effect and wavelet outliers due to the regularization on the adjacent voxels, as shown in Fig. 2. Based on the above observation, we propose a fast non-local tensor total variation (NL-TTV) algorithm to overcome the above limitations of the local TTV method.

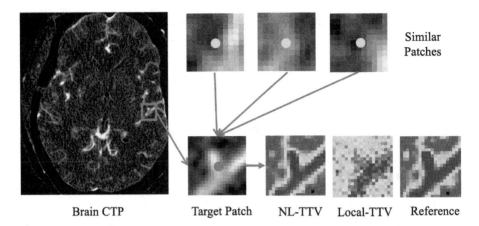

Similar Patches

Brain CTP   Target Patch   NL-TTV   Local-TTV   Reference

Fig. 2. Illustration of the non-local tensor total variation principle in a 2D image. The NL-TTV regularization term for voxel i (red dot) is a weighted summation of the difference between voxel i and the most similar voxels (yellow dots) in the search window with width W (red box). The weight $w(i, j)$ depends on the patches around the voxels. Compared to local-TTV, which only considers the 4-connected local neighborhood, NL-TTV preserves the accuracy and contrast of the vascular structure with higher fidelity of the reference patch. The actual NL-TTV regularization is imposed on 4D spatio-temporal flow-scaled residue impulse functions across different slices and time points. (Color figure online)

2.2 Non-local Tensor Total Variation Deconvolution

First introduced by [13], non-local total variation has been studied to address the limitations of conventional total variation model, including the blocky effect, the missing of the small edges and the lack of long-range information sharing [14–16]. It has also been applied to 4D computed tomography [17] and magnetic resonance imaging reconstruction [18]. This work is the first attempt to integrate non-local tensor total variation with the spatio-temporal deconvolution problem in 4D CTP.

The non-local tensor total variation regularizer links each voxel in the volume with the long-range voxels using a weighted function. For every voxel i, instead of computing the forward finite difference on the 4-connected neighbors, we search in a neighborhood window $N(i)$ with window size W, and minimize the weighted differences between the target voxel and voxels in the window. Specifically, the non-local tensor total variation can be formulated as:

$$\|K\|_{NL-TTV} = \sum_i \sqrt{\sum_j (K(i) - K(j))^2 w(i, j)} \qquad (3)$$

Here $K(i)$ denotes the value of flow-scaled residue impulse function K at spatio-temporal voxel i, and $w(i, j)$ is a similarity function between the voxel i and j. The higher the similarity between the voxels i and j, the higher the weight function $w(i, j)$. We use an exponential function of the patches surround the two voxels to model their similarity

$$w(i,j) = \frac{1}{Z(i)} e^{-\frac{\|K(P_i) - K(P_j)\|_2^2}{\sigma^2}} \tag{4}$$

where Z is a normalization factor, with $Z(i) = \sum_j w(i, j)$ and σ is a filter parameter that controls the shape of the similarity function. P_i is a small patch around voxel i with radius d. In this way, when two patches are identical or similar, the weight w will be close to 1; when the two patches are very different, the weight w will approach 0. Non-local total variation has shown superior performance signal reconstruction and denoising [14,15], and by fusing it with the temporal convolution model, we get

$$K_{NL-TTV} = \underset{K \in \mathbb{R}^{T \times N}}{\arg \min} (\frac{1}{2} \|AK - C\|_2^2 + \|K\|_{NL-TTV}) \tag{5}$$

The non-local tensor total variation searches for the similar patches in a larger window instead of the adjacent 4-connected neighbors in the local TTV. In this way, the similar tissue patterns of the same tissue types in the long-range regions of the brain can assist to reduce the artifact and noise in the deconvolution process. This allow the NL-TTV to deconvolve the low-dose CTP volume using long-range and global dependency by removing the noise without distorting the salient structures, as shown in Fig. 2.

It is worthy to note that because the voxel i is any voxel in the spatio-temporal domain of the flow-scaled residue impulse function $K \in \mathbb{R}^{T \times N}$, the NL-TTV is searching the similar patches in the spatio-temporal domain, which includes the multiple slices in the axial direction and the various time points in the temporal sequences.

2.3 Efficient Optimization and Implementation

We implement this algorithm by MATLAB and C++ using mex in MATLAB 2013a environment (MathWorks Inc, Natick, MA) and Windows 8 operating system with 8 Intel Core i5 and 32 GB RAM.

Notations: Let's define some parameters first. Let N be the total number of voxels in the entire volume. W be the search window size for the similar voxels around voxel i. d is the radius of the patch around the voxel. N_b is the number of similar voxels chosen to regularize the voxel i in order to speed up the computation. m is the dimension of the spatio-temporal tensor. σ is the Gaussian parameter to control the shape of the similarity function.

In this work, for a 2D slice in the brain CTP data of 512×512 voxels, $120\,s$ of scanning duration, $W = 5$ voxels, $d = 4$ voxels, $N_b = 15$, $\sigma = 0.5$. $m = 4$ because the flow-scaled residue impulse functions are spatio-temporal tensor with 4 dimensions.

Brute-Force Search: The non-local tensor total variation has a higher time complexity compared to the local TTV. For each voxel i in the volume, we need to calculate the patch difference between the target voxel and every other voxel in the search window. Then we rank all the patch differences in voxel i's search window in an ascending order, and pick up the first N_b patches for optimizing the value of i.

The time complexity of the brutal force non-local TTV is $O(N \cdot ((2W+1)(2d+1))^m + N \cdot (2W + 1)^m \log(N_b))$. For the parameters above, the computational time reaches up to nearly *10 hours*, which is unrealistic in clinical applications.

Fast Nearest Neighbor Search: An efficient method to compute the intensity difference between two patches is used to accelerate the non-local TTV is needed. Specifically, at each offset $w = (w_x, w_y, w_z, w_t)$ in the search window W, a new matrix D of the same size to the brain volume is created to precompute the patch differences, with $D_w = \sum_i (K(i + w) - K(i))^2$. This matrix keeps the sum of the squared differences from the upper left corner to the current voxel. When computing the differences between the two patches at location j and offset w, we only need to compute the value $D(j_x + d, j_y + d) - D(j_x + d, j_y) - D(j_x, j_y + d) + D(j_x, j_y)$. This accelerating method to find the nearest neighbors reduced the time complexity to $O(N \cdot (2W + 1)^m + \log(N_b))$. The space complexity is $N \cdot (2W + 1)^m$.

Efficient Optimization Algorithm: Due to the relatively slow update in the non-local TTV term, we propose a fast NLTTV algorithm to optimize the objective function in Eq. (5), as outlined in Algorithm 1. In the iterative optimization, K is initialized with zero first, and updated using steepest gradient descent from the temporal convolution model. Then it is further updated using the NL-TTV regularizer with accelerated step. In the accelerated step, instead of alternating between the non-local TTV term and the temporal convolution term once each iteration, we update the non-local TTV term *fewer* times than updating the temporal convolution term, which has shown sufficient accuracy in the experimental results.

Parallel Computing: The intrinsic nature of non-local TTV algorithm allows for multi-threading and parallel computing on the multi-core clusters or grids. We divide the entire brain volume into sub-volumes, with each of them processed by one processor. The patch difference computation for every voxel i and the weight calculation for all the voxels after selecting the top N_b neighbors can be paralleled.

3   Experiments

Experimental Setting: The goal of our proposed method is to accurately estimate the hemodynamic parameters in low-dose CTP by robust deconvolution (Fig. 3). Due to the ethical issues and potential health risk associated with scanning the same subject twice under different radiation doses, we follow the experimental setting in [9] to simulate low-dose CTP data at 15 mAs by adding correlated Gaussian noise with standard deviation of $\sigma = 25$ [19]. Please note that low-dose simulated is a widely adopted method CT algorithm evaluation

Algorithm 1. The framework of NL-TTV algorithm.

Input: $K^0 = r^1 = 0$, $t^1 = C = 0$, τ
Output: Flow-scaled residue functions $K \in \mathbb{R}^{T \times N_1 \times N_2 \times N_3}$.
for $n = 1, 2, \ldots, N$ **do**
  $C = C + 1$
  (1) Steepest gradient descent $K_g = r^n + s^{n+1} A^T (C - A r^n)$
  where $s^{n+1} = \frac{vec(Q)^T vec(Q)}{vec(AQ)^T vec(AQ)}$, $Q \equiv A^T (A r^n - C)$, $vec(\cdot)$ vectorizes a matrix
  (2) Proximal map:
  if $C = \tau$ (*Acceleration Step*) **then**
    $K^n = \text{prox}_\gamma (2\|K\|_{NL-TTV})(fold(K_g))$, $C = 0$
    where $\text{prox}_\rho(g)(x) := \underset{u}{\arg\min} \left\{ g(u) + \frac{1}{2\rho}\|u - x\|^2 \right\}$, and $fold(K_g)$ folds the
    matrix K_g into a tensor $\tilde{K} \in \mathbb{R}^{T \times N_1 \times N_2 \times N_3}$.
  end if
  (3) Update t, r $t^{n+1} = (1 + \sqrt{1 + 4(t^n)^2})/2$, $r^{n+1} = K^n + ((t^n - 1)/t^{n+1})(K^n - K^{n-1})$
end for

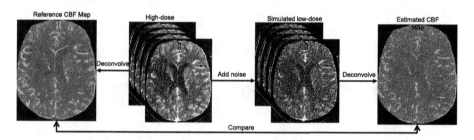

Fig. 3. Simulation of low-dose CTP data from high-dose CTP data and the evaluation framework

in the medical field [20, 21]. The deconvolution methods are evaluated on the simulated low-dose CTP data. The quality of the CBF maps of all methods are evaluated by comparing with the reference maps using peak signal-to-noise ratio (PSNR). While PSNR may not be the best evaluation metric for the clinical dataset, it is an objective reflection of the fidelity between the perfusion maps of the low-dose and the normal dose data.

Our method is evaluated on a clinical dataset of 10 subjects admitted to the Weill Cornell Medical College with mean age (range) of 53 (42–63) years and four of them had brain deficits due to aneurysmal subarachnoid hemorrhage (aSAH) or ischemic stroke, and the rest were normal. CTP images were collected with a standard protocol using GE Lightspeed Pro-16 scanners (General Electric Medical Systems, Milwaukee, WI) with cine 4i scanning mode and 60 s acquisition at 1 rotation per second, 0.5 s per sample, using 80 kVp and 190 mA. Four 5-mm-thick sections with pixel spacing of 0.43 mm between centers of columns and rows were assessed at the level of the third ventricle and the basal ganglia, yielding a spatio-temporal tensor of $512 \times 512 \times 4 \times 118$ where there are 4 slices and 119 temporal samples. Approximately 45 mL of nonionic iodinated contrast was administered intravenously at 5 mL/s using a power injector with a 5 s delay.

Results: Figure 4 shows the representative CBF maps of a subject with brain deficits in the right hemisphere (upper panel) and a normal subject (lower panel). For each subject, from left to right shows the reference map, the low-dose maps of standard singular value decomposition (sSVD) [22], block-circulant singular value decomposition (bSVD) [23], Tikhonov [24], local tensor total variation (TTV) [9], and our proposed non-local TTV (NL-TTV).

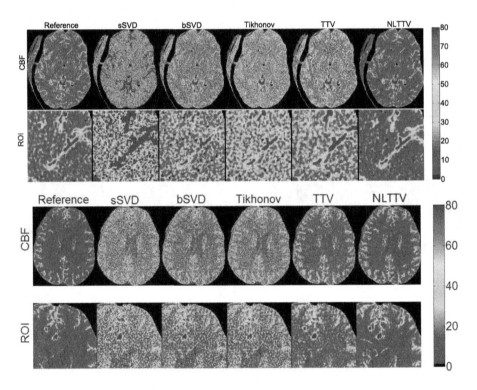

Fig. 4. Results from a subject with right frontoparietal craniotomy due to ischemia in the right anterior cerebral artery (RACA) and right middle cerebral artery (RMCA) territories (upper panel), and a normal subject (lower panel). In each panel, the first row is the entire CBF map and the second row is the closeup view of selected regions.

The entire brain image and the close-up views demonstrate significant improvement in the overall accuracy and preservation of the delicate anatomical structures using the non-local TTV method for both the deficit and the normal subjects. sSVD tends to severely over-estimate CBF, while SVD-based methods also over-estimate perfusion parameters. TTV performs better than the SVD-based methods in preserving the quantitative accuracy and the contrast resolution between different tissue classes. However, TTV still over-estimates the CBF value, and the capillaries in the close-up view are dilated due to the local smoothing using the tensor total variation regularization. On the contrary, NL-TTV overcomes both issues. The quantitative accuracy of the perfusion maps improve significantly, and more noticeably, the small vessels and capillaries in the brain are precisely preserved without dilation or rupture, as we can observe in the local TTV results.

Quantitative results on the images of 10 subjects are shown in Fig. 5(a). Our proposed method significantly outperforms all other comparison methods ($p < 0.05$). The algorithm converges within 10 iterations (Fig. 5(b)).

The running time of the entire CTP data of one subject is around 30 min, after our accelerated optimization. Since the algorithm is implemented in MAT-LAB platform and run on a single PC desktop, grid or cluster computing is expected to speed up the experiments.

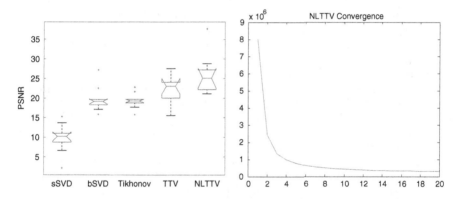

Fig. 5. (a) Boxplot of PSNR and SSIM for the 10 clinical subjects. The proposed NL-TTV method significantly outperforms all other comparison methods ($p < 0.05$). (b) Convergence curve of the cost function for NL-TTV algorithm.

4 Conclusion

In this paper, we proposed an efficient non-local tensor total variation method for low-dose CT perfusion deconvolution. The long-range and global similarities of the same tissue classes in the brain structure are leveraged to stabilize the spatio-temporal residue functions. The overall quantitative accuracy is significantly improved with the delicate anatomical structures such as capillaries well preserved to assist clinical diagnosis. Fast optimization and implementation schemes are presented to reduce the time complexity and computational cost. Extensive evaluations with comparison to the existing algorithms, including sSVD, bSVD, Tikhonov and local TTV, demonstrate the superior performance of the non-local TTV method in low-dose deconvolution and perfusion parameter estimation.

References

1. Saito, N., Kudo, K., Sasaki, T., Uesugi, M., Koshino, K., Miyamoto, M., Suzuki, S.: Realization of reliable cerebral-blood-flow maps from low-dose CT perfusion images by statistical noise reduction using nonlinear diffusion filtering. Radiol. Phys. Technol. **1**(1), 62–74 (2008)
2. Mendrik, A.M., Vonken, E., van Ginneken, B., de Jong, H.W., Riordan, A., van Seeters, T., Smit, E.J., Viergever, M.A., Prokop, M.: Tips bilateral noise reduction in 4d CT perfusion scans produceshigh-quality cerebral blood flow maps. Phys. Med. Biol. **56**(13), 3857 (2011)
3. Tian, Z., Jia, X., Yuan, K., Pan, T., Jiang, S.B.: Low-dose CT reconstruction via edge-preserving total variation regularization. Phys. Med. Biol. **56**(18), 5949 (2011)
4. Ma, J., Huang, J., Feng, Q., Zhang, H., Lu, H., Liang, Z., Chen, W.: Low-dose computed tomography image restoration using previous normal-dose scan. Med. Phys. **38**, 5713 (2011)
5. Supanich, M., Tao, Y., Nett, B., Pulfer, K., Hsieh, J., Turski, P., Mistretta, C., Rowley, H., Chen, G.H.: Radiation dose reduction in time-resolved CT angiography using highly constrained back projection reconstruction. Phys. Med. Biol. **54**(14), 4575 (2009)
6. He, L., Orten, B., Do, S., Karl, W.C., Kambadakone, A., Sahani, D.V., Pien, H.: A spatio-temporal deconvolution method to improve perfusion CT quantification. IEEE Trans. Med. Imaging **29**(5), 1182–1191 (2010)
7. Fang, R., Chen, T., Sanelli, P.C.: Towards robust deconvolution of low-dose perfusion CT: sparse perfusion deconvolution using online dictionary learning. Med. Image Anal. **17**(4), 417–428 (2013)
8. Fang, R., Karlsson, K., Chen, T., Sanelli, P.C.: Improving low-dose blood-brain barrier permeability quantification using sparse high-dose induced prior for patlak model. Med. Image Anal. **18**(6), 866–880 (2014)
9. Fang, R., Zhang, S., Chen, T., Sanelli, P.: Robust low-dose CT perfusion deconvolution via tensor total-variation regularization. IEEE Trans. Med. Imaging **34**(7), 1533–1548 (2015)
10. Yu, Y., Zhang, S., Li, K., Metaxas, D., Axel, L.: Deformable models with sparsity constraints for cardiac motion analysis. Med. Image Anal. **18**(6), 927–937 (2014)
11. Zhang, S., Zhan, Y., Dewan, M., Huang, J., Metaxas, D.N., Zhou, X.S.: Towards robust and effective shape modeling: sparse shape composition. Med. Image Anal. **16**(1), 265–277 (2012)
12. Fang, R., Sanelli, P.C., Zhang, S., Chen, T.: Tensor total-variation regularized deconvolution for efficient low-dose CT perfusion. In: Golland, P., Hata, N., Barillot, C., Hornegger, J., Howe, R. (eds.) MICCAI 2014, Part I. LNCS, vol. 8673, pp. 154–161. Springer, Heidelberg (2014)
13. Sawatzky, A.: (Nonlocal) Total Variation in Medical Imaging, Ph.D. Thesis
14. Zhang, X., Burger, M., Bresson, X., Osher, S.: Bregmanized nonlocal regularization for deconvolution and sparse reconstruction. SIAM J. Imaging Sci. **3**(3), 253–276 (2010)
15. Mignotte, M.: A non-local regularization strategy for image deconvolution. Pattern Recogn. Lett. **29**(16), 2206–2212 (2008)
16. Elmoataz, A., Lezoray, O., Bougleux, S.: Nonlocal discrete regularization on weighted graphs: a framework for image and manifold processing. IEEE Trans. Image Process. **17**(7), 1047–1060 (2008)

17. Jia, X., Lou, Y., Dong, B., Tian, Z., Jiang, S.: 4D computed tomography reconstruction from few-projection data via temporal non-local regularization. In: Jiang, T., Navab, N., Pluim, J.P.W., Viergever, M.A. (eds.) MICCAI 2010, Part I. LNCS, vol. 6361, pp. 143–150. Springer, Heidelberg (2010)

18. Huang, J., Yang, F.: Compressed magnetic resonance imaging based on wavelet sparsity and nonlocal total variation. In: 2012 9th IEEE International Symposium on Biomedical Imaging (ISBI), pp. 968–971. IEEE (2012)

19. Britten, A., Crotty, M., Kiremidjian, H., Grundy, A., Adam, E.: The addition of computer simulated noise to investigate radiation dose and image quality in images with spatial correlation of statistical noise: an example application to X-ray CT of the brain. Br. J. Radiol. **77**, 323–328 (2014)

20. Juluru, K., Shih, J., Raj, A., Comunale, J., Delaney, H., Greenberg, E., Hermann, C., Liu, Y., Hoelscher, A., Al-Khori, N., et al.: Effects of increased image noise on image quality and quantitative interpretation in brain CT perfusion. Am. J. Neuroradiol. **34**(8), 1506–1512 (2013)

21. Frush, D.P., Slack, C.C., Hollingsworth, C.L., Bisset, G.S., Donnelly, L.F., Hsieh, J., Lavin-Wensell, T., Mayo, J.R.: Computer-simulated radiation dose reduction for abdominal multidetector CT of pediatric patients. Am. J. Roentgenol. **179**(5), 1107–1113 (2002)

22. Østergaard, L., Weisskoff, R.M., Chesler, D.A., Gyldensted, C., Rosen, B.R.: High resolution measurement of cerebral blood flow using intravascular tracer bolus passages. Part I: Mathematical approach and statistical analysis. Magn. Reson. Med. **36**(5), 715–725 (1996)

23. Wittsack, H.J., Wohlschläger, A.M., Ritzl, E., Kleiser, R., Cohnen, M., Seitz, R., Mödder, U.: CT-perfusion imaging of the human brain: advanced deconvolution analysis using circulant singular value decomposition. Comput. Med. Imaging Graph. **32**(1), 67–77 (2008)

24. Fieselmann, A., Kowarschik, M., Ganguly, A., Hornegger, J., Fahrig, R.: Deconvolution-based CT and MR brain perfusion measurement: theoretical model revisited and practical implementation details. J. Biomed. Imaging **2011**, 14 (2011)

Author Index

Printed in the United States
By Bookmasters